THE
PROSTATE
CANCER
BOOK

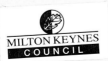

THE
PROSTATE
CANCER
BOOK

Professor Jonathan Waxman

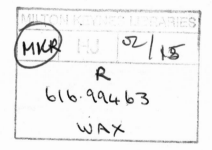

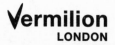

Vermilion
LONDON

1 3 5 7 9 10 8 6 4 2

Copyright © Jonathan Waxman 2001

Jonathan Waxman has asserted his moral right to be identified
as the author of this work in accordance with the Copyright, Designs
and Patents Act 1988.

First published in 2002 by Vermilion,
an imprint of Ebury Press, Random House,
20 Vauxhall Bridge Road, London SW1V 2SA
www.randomhouse.co.uk

Random House Australia (Pty) Limited
20 Alfred Street, Milsons Point, Sydney,
New South Wales 2061, Australia

Random House New Zealand Limited
18 Poland Road, Glenfield, Auckland 10, New Zealand

Random House South Africa (Pty) Limited
Endulini, 5a Jubilee Road, Parktown 2193, South Africa

The Random House Group Limited Reg. No. 954009

Papers used by Vermilion are natural, recyclable products made from wood
grown in sustainable forests.

Printed and bound in Great Britain by Mackays of Chatham plc, Chatham, Kent

A CIP catalogue record for this book is available from the British Library.

ISBN 0 09 185712 0

This book is written as a source of information only. The information
in this book should by no means be considered a substitute for
the advice, decisions or judgment of the reader's physician or other
professional advisor. No decisions regarding diagnosis, prognosis or
treatment should be made on the basis of this book alone. The author
and the publisher disclaim responsibility for any adverse affects
arising from the use or application of the information contained
herein. No real patient names have been used in this book.

Contents

Acknowledgements

I should like to acknowledge the contributions of Kay McCauley, who told me that I just had to write this book, Chris Hiley, who helped with comments that made me think again about my words and their interpretation, Sandie Coward, who typed and proofread, Keya d'Sa, who produced the art work, and Russ Hargreaves who pointed to the need for a proper patient information book. I thank my patients, for all that they have shown me.

Introduction

For a long time prostate cancer simply was not talked about. Now, some thirty years after the example set by the women's movement in successfully bringing breast cancer to the attention of the wider public, prostate cancer has finally come out of the closet.

Why was prostate cancer surrounded by silence for so long? Prostate cancer sat in the closet because it affected men and occupied a part of the body that is was not quite polite to talk about. Prostate cancer used to be very much a disease of older men: it affects a generation of men with an average age of approximately 72. These were primarily men who had gone through the Second World War and who were used to shouldering responsibility for their families. They did not want to become a burden to the family they loved, and so they dealt with their disease privately, without causing a fuss. A second reason is the area of the body affected by the disease, an area obliquely referred to by this older generation of men as their 'private parts'. The prostate gland is important in sexual function, and prostate malfunction presents urinary symptoms, symptoms that used to be – and to a great extent still are – taboo in polite company. Furthermore, the condition of the prostate gland is assessed via the rectum. In a very real sense, prostate cancer was considered to be a private affair. For these reasons, it wasn't talked about.

But now the situation has changed. With a new generation of men, a generation that is perhaps a little less reticent about coming forward, the subject of prostate cancer has now moved out into the public domain. Men are more willing to talk openly about their health. They are also becoming better informed about men's health issues in general.

Much of this change has been brought about by women, because women are more medicalised than men. That is to say, they have had greater experience of medical practice as a result of their need to deal with contraception, their contact with the medical profession when they have had their babies, visits to the GP for screening tests for cervical or breast cancer, and the fact that they tend to be the medical carers for the family, shouldering responsibility for the health of their babies, their children and their men. From my experience, it is generally women who accompany their men to the doctor's when their symptoms have become too significant to be ignored, take them through their hospital visits, sit with them in the consulting room and remember the conversations that take place in the course of diagnosis and treatment.

Working together, men and women have successfully raised public awareness about the importance of prostate cancer. And it is an important illness: prostate cancer is currently the second most common cause of male cancer deaths in the West, and death rates have trebled over the last thirty years. Now, on both sides of the Atlantic, research funding has increased and governments are actively engaged in supporting both research and people with this cancer. Heightened public awareness means that more and more men are presenting themselves voluntarily for screening for prostate cancer.

About This Book

I work as an oncologist, and have over the years carried out clinical and laboratory research into prostate cancer. I have written this book for people with prostate cancer, and for their families and friends. A diagnosis of prostate cancer is a potentially distressing time for all concerned, so in this book I try to explain the possible psychological and emotional reactions you may experience, both at the time of diagnosis and while following a course of treatment. I hope that the practical information about the causes, diagnosis and treatment contained within these pages will help you to feel better informed when faced with decisions and choices.

Before you read this book, I should point out that the efficacy of a particular course of treatment is arrived at from an analysis of the results of clinical trials. Ongoing research means that treatments are in a constant state of evolution, and so in some areas of prostate cancer management the advantages of one type of treatment over another have not yet been clinically proven. As a result, opinions sometimes differ as to which might be the best course of treatment for the individual patient. In those areas where opinions are known to differ, I shall try to give you the fullest possible picture so that you know exactly what options are open to you.

At all stages of the diagnostic and treatment procedures, I advise you to discuss things fully with your physician – remember, they're on your side. Towards the back of the book you will find some examples of the sort of questions to ask them. You will also find the names and address of support organisations as well as sources of further information.

CHAPTER ONE

What is the Prostate
and What Are the Conditions Effecting It?

The prostate is the shape and size of a walnut and is located low down in the pelvis, at the base of the bladder. It starts life as a tiny gland, whose growth and development during infant life are influenced by the principal male hormone, testosterone, and a number of other hormones produced by the pituitary gland. The pituitary, which sits in the centre of the brain, is the main hormone-producing organ of the body – growth hormone, prolactins (which in women help the manufacture of milk) and to a lesser extent thyroid hormones are all important in the growth of the prostate gland.

In adolescence the gland enlarges further, while growth occurring within the prostate itself leads to the development of microscopic glands which produce the prostatic secretion called *prostate specific antigen* (PSA). This fluid, which is rich in sugar and enzymes, has an important role to play in sexual activity. Sperm produced in the testicles drains through a series of tubes called the epididymis, then along the inguinal canal before passing deep into the pelvis to meet the prostate. Here PSA, which drains from the prostatic glands along a collection of tiny tubes (prostatic ducts), is released into the sperm at the moment of orgasm. The sperm is nourished by this sugar-rich fluid and kept alive for its journey into the outside world.

The main function of PSA is to clear away the residual matter left within the prostatic ducts after orgasm – if left alone, this debris would solidify and block them. The action by which the enzymes in PSA dissolve and remove this debris is termed 'protease activity'. In other words, the enzymatic activity of PSA keeps the system clean. The level of PSA normally present in the bloodstream reflects the activity and health of the prostate gland. This can be measured by a PSA test.

Prostate growth continues with the years, and enlargement of the gland may be such that it can cause significant difficulties. In particular, the gland's physical location may lead to problems with urination. When you urinate, urine flows from

A virtual section through the body showing the prostate and surrounding structures.

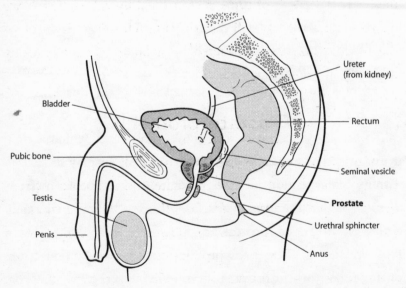

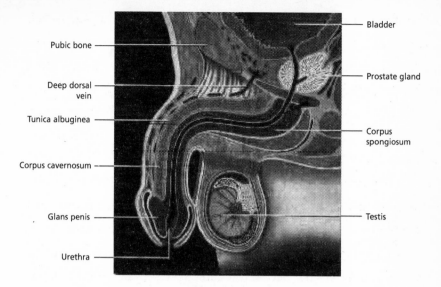

Pubic bone

Deep dorsal vein

Tunica albuginea

Corpus cavernosum

Glans penis

Urethra

Bladder

Prostate gland

Corpus spongiosum

Testis

A more detailed section of the body showing the prostate and surrounding area.

the bladder along a tube called the urethra, which passes through the centre of the prostate before leaving the body via the penis. The flow of urine is controlled by valves, which are opened and closed at will on urination. However, the neck of the bladder may be obstructed by a large prostate, causing difficulty in urine flow.

Prostate problems

Benign Prostatic Hypertrophy (BPH)

Benign enlargement of the prostate, otherwise known as *benign prostatic hypertrophy*, or BPH for short, is the most common cause of prostate problems. It is a condition of normal ageing. The prostate simply becomes larger. Treatments are aimed at limiting its size. These may take the form

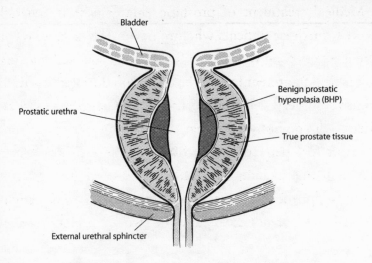

Bladder

Benign prostatic
hyperplasia (BHP)

Prostatic urethra

True prostate tissue

External urethral sphincter

A cross section through the prostate showing its relationship to neighbouring structures.

of a surgical operation or medical treatment to reverse the effects of the hormones controlling the prostate's growth. The surgical treatment of BPH is known as *transurethral prostatectomy*, or TURP. In this operation a tube is inserted through the penis along the urethra to clear away the physical obstruction.

Because the enlargement of the prostate is a process that takes place over many years, medical treatment of BPH is generally less effective than surgery. Medical treatments for benign enlargement will take a considerable period of time to improve urinary symptoms. It is estimated that over a period of approximately one year, 30% of patients will have a 30% improvement of their urinary symptoms with medical treatments. A TURP will lead to an improvement in nearly all patients.

Medical treatment of prostatic enlargement is generally reserved for those patients who are not fit for surgery. Where there is a very long waiting list for surgery, your GP may give you medical treatment to ease the condition during the wait for definitive surgery. Medical treatments are also reserved for patients who do not want to have surgery but would like some treatment for their condition. Many of these treatments are hormonal and include the LHRH agonists and finasteride. Dietary supplements such as Saw Palmetto have some activity. Although we are not clear how this works, it does have an effect.

Prostatitis

Prostatitis is an inflammation of the prostate gland. It can be caused by infection or may sometimes be acquired as a result of sexual activity. Prostatitis is frequently very uncomfortable: symptoms include significant pain, usually with a temperature and often with frequency of urination. Treatment is with antibiotics and may be required for more than two weeks. In some cases these may need to be administered intravenously. Prostatitis can unfortunately be a recurring problem and may require many courses of antibiotics before it is finally eliminated from the body.

Prostate Cancer

Prostate cancer can vary from the most benign of conditions to a significant illness. Uncommon in younger men, the frequency with which cancer affects the prostate gland increases with age. In fact a small spot of prostate cancer is very common in older men, occurring in up to 80% of 80-year olds who, having died from a cause other than prostate cancer, have had their prostate examined at post-mortem. These little spots of prostate cancer – or *foci*, as they are called – occur in 70% of 70-year olds, 60% of 60-year olds and 50% of 50-year olds. The relationship between these spots of cancer and the development of a malignant growth is as yet unknown.

An even more benign variant is termed *prostatic intraepithelial neoplasia,* or PIN. There is controversy whether PIN

A microscopic view of the prostate in low and high power magnification to show PIN.

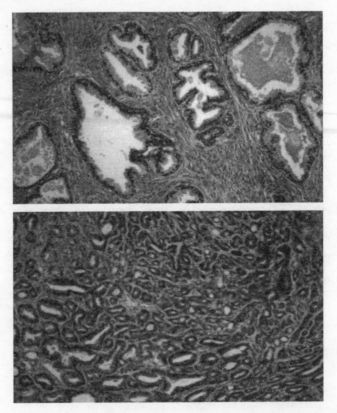

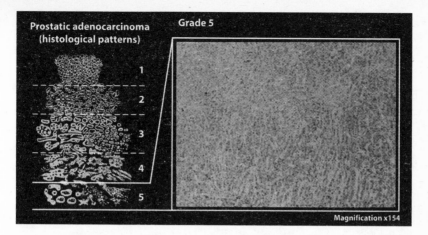

Undifferentiated tumour. Minimal glandular differentiation. Diffusely infiltrating anaplastic cells.

is significant or not. Some doctors regard PIN as being the equivalent of the female conditions in breast and cervical cancer which lead to the development of an invasive tumour. However, the great majority of doctors have no such view and remain unconvinced as to whether or not PIN has any relationship with overt prostate cancer. PIN may cause no symptoms and may be completely benign, and this is in contrast to the 'equivalents' in the breast and cervix. If you are diagnosed as having PIN, you should be reassured that hopefully there will be no progression to an invasive cancer. You will also be advised to keep an annual check on the situation by PSA testing and continued medical follow-up.

Prostate cancer may cause problems with urination. These can be due either to the physical enlargement of the gland or to the invasion of the prostatic urethral valves so that they become rigid and are unable to open and shut under normal control. This will cause significant symptoms, making it very difficult to pass urine normally. The bladder enlarges, and may do so to such an extent that in the end it becomes impossible to pass urine. This can cause considerable pain and requires admission to hospital for catheterisation to relieve the obstruction. Symptoms are relieved within a few moments of passing the catheter.

Advances in treatment mean that a diagnosis of prostate cancer need no longer trigger our worst fears. Indeed, for many men, prostate cancer is a relatively indolent disease – a cancer that causes no significant problems in their lives. A significant number of others are cured of their illness, whilst a further proportion may have their symptoms eased for a significant period of time. In any event, survival is a probability not a remote possibility.

In the next chapter we shall look at the causes of prostate cancer and at the factors that can increase your susceptibility to it. We shall also look at some of the things you can do, if you are free of the disease, to reduce the risk of developing it.

CHAPTER TWO

What Causes Prostate Cancer?

One of the first things many patients do when they receive a diagnosis of cancer is to look to their lives to try to establish what it is that has caused their illness. They often ask themselves, 'Is it me, or is it something I've done?'. They may even ask themselves whether they have got cancer because of their genes or because of their particular lifestyle.

Your Genes

We are what we are as a result of the genetic load we inherit from our parents, our grandparents and all the generations that have preceded us. In recent years there have been many analyses of the possible role of genetics in the development of cancers. A number of studies have also looked at the family histories of patients with prostate cancer to ascertain whether any of their relatives have developed the disease. In these studies details of the patients' family histories have been put together and extensively analysed to establish the significance of inheritance as a possible cause of prostate cancer.

One of the largest studies was carried out in Canada at the

Laval University and published in 1995. 7,277 men with prostate cancer were questioned, and a family history of prostate cancer was obtained in only a small number of cases. Just 103 men had brothers who had developed prostate cancer, and 56 men had fathers who had had the illness, implying that genes are not significant in the development of prostate cancer. That is, out of a sample of over 7,000 men, only 159 had a positive family history. This is very unlike the situation for many other cancers. The evidence produced by the study shows that if your father was affected by the disease, the relative risk of your getting prostate cancer is increased 1.2-fold. Should a brother be affected, the risk is increased 2.6-fold. Although this increase may seem significant, it is important to note that this risk only applies to a very small number of men: out of over 7,000, only 2% had a family history of prostate cancer.

The results of this study clearly imply that our genes have very little to do with the development of prostate cancer. This fact comes as a relief for many men who receive a positive diagnosis, because they know that the risk of passing the disease on to their sons is not significantly increased.

There is a theory that an underlying genetic propensity to cancer can be sparked by exposure to an environmental agent, whether chemical or viral, and this causes the cancer to develop. This theory has many protagonists. However, as I will show you, *with prostate cancer all the evidence seems to point to environmental causes for the disease.*

Your Race and Age

The incidence of prostate cancer varies enormously around the world. It is unusual in the Far East and in rural areas of Africa. Some clues as to the causes of prostate cancer have been provided by studies of migrating populations. One such study involved migrants from Japan and China who had settled in the United States and Hawaii in the mid-19th century. These communities were relatively insular and there was little inter-marriage. Over the generations that succeeded the first wave of immigration there have been significant changes in the incidence of prostate cancer. The first generation of migrants were called the Issei, and the second generation the Nissei. For every 10 Caucasian Americans dying from prostate cancer, there was only 1 Japanese death in the initial migrant generation: a ratio of 10:1. This ratio changed to 5:1 for the Issei and to 1.5:1 for the Nissei. Given that there was such little inter-marriage, one looks for other factors that may be causing the increased incidence of the development of prostate cancer. Where these migrants are concerned, *the only thing that has really changed is their environment.*

In the case of African-Americans the disease is even more significant than in white populations. As the following table clearly shows, the risk of African-Americans developing prostate cancer is so much greater that it is similar to that of white Americans of much greater age. We have no idea why this should be, although it is possible that there are complex biochemical differences at the level of DNA between Afro-Caribbeans and Caucasians involving what are termed 'tri-nucleotide repeats' on the Y chromosome.

Prostate cancer age-specific incidence rates

Age	Japan	San Francisco (White)	San Francisco (Black)
		cases per 100,000 population	
40–44	0.5	1.5	2.3
45–59	0.4	5.4	10.8
50–54	1.0	14.3	62.1
55–59	3.2	64.8	174
60–64	8.3	153	290
65–69	27.5	286	418
70–74	51.1	484	1007
75–79	65.4	721	1009
80–84	80.3	909	1486
85 plus	110.5	938	865

National Cancer Institute Monograph 53. 1979, 149

This table describes the rate of prostate cancer in different populations, where groups of similar numbers of patients are compared.

Prostate cancer is an illness of older men. That is, the incidence of prostate cancer increases almost exponentially as men age, and this can be seen in the table above. This is yet further evidence that prostate cancer is caused by environmental factors, because the environmental risk factors accumulate as you grow older. *The longer you live, the more environmental risk factors you will have been exposed to.*

Your Sexual Activity and Married State

As prostate cancer affects a gland that is uniquely under the control of male hormones, it would seem logical that there should be some relationship between the development of the disease and the levels of male hormones in the blood and sexual activity.

The effects of sexual activity are difficult to document because it is hard to measure sexual activity objectively, and even more difficult to make comparisons between different populations. However, evidence first came to light about 20 years ago on the possible importance of sexual activity in the development of prostate cancer. Patients with prostate cancer were found to have an increased likelihood of having had a sexually transmitted disease, to have had more sexual partners and possibly to have a greater libido than either men without prostate cancer or men with benign enlargement of the prostate gland (BPH). The study suggests that married men are at greater risk of developing prostate cancer, as are divorcees or widowers. Single men are the least likely to develop the disease. The evidence produced in this study, comes from an analysis of a small number of people and was not considered to have validity. Surprisingly, more evidence emerged in 2001 confirming the possible link between sex and prostate cancer, linking numbers of sexual partners and lack of condom use with an increased risk of prostate cancer. So there may be something in the story.

Circulating levels of the male hormone testosterone have been measured in patients with prostate cancer and compared and contrasted with levels in normal patients and in patients with benign enlargement of the gland. For many years it was thought that, in comparison to these controls, patients with prostate cancer had similar levels of the male hormone.

However, recent evidence would seem to point to slightly higher levels of testosterone in prostate cancer patients than in normal men. This point has been debated considerably and is by no means medical fact. But as we shall see later, the control of testosterone levels is an important factor in the hormonal treatment of prostate cancer.

Although there is a very small body of opinion that suggests that prostate cancer may be related to sexual activity, the evidence is contentious and the risk is certainly a very small component in the development of the disease. In view of this it would be senseless to burden yourself with any sort of guilt about past relationships. Nor would it be of any value to disturb a loving relationship on the off chance that doing so could decrease your risk of developing carcinoma of the prostate.

Diet

As the old adage says, 'we are what we eat', and there is certainly an increasing public awareness of the overwhelming significance of diet in the development of many diseases. For instance, it has been shown that heart disease is linked to the consumption of animal fat, and colorectal cancer to diets that are low in fibre. Both of these diseases, which are associated with the modern high-fat, low-fibre Western diet, are virtually unknown in the rural Third World.

It has been known for the last 20 years that prostate cancer has a significant dietary basis. Indeed, there may be additional protection against cancer from specific diets. The China study has shown that consumers of diets that are rich in yellow beans are further protected from the development of prostate cancer. The reduction in risk is nearly five fold, and so very important. In 1999, an exhaustive prospective study of dietary risk factors was published. Called the Netherlands Cohorts Study, this was an analysis of the diets and medical fates of over 56,000 men. The men, aged between 55 and 69 years, were followed over a period of nearly seven years and during this time assessments made of what they ate. During the period of the study 642 men (1.5%) developed prostate cancer. Those who had consumed significant amounts of cured meat and milk products were at much greater risk of developing prostate cancer.

There is overwhelming statistical evidence that cancer occurs at half the rate in vegetarians that it does in meat-eating omnivores. However, it is not known whether this is due to additives such as preservatives, antibiotics and colouring agents or whether it is the consumption of meat itself which is the cause. It is thought that a group of chemicals called phyto-oestrogens, which are female hormone-like chemicals present in plants, are responsible for the protective effect of a vegetarian diet. It may well be that all that is required in this matter is a little sense, and sense quite remarkably fits with the UK Government's health guidelines recommendation that we consume at least five portions of fruit and vegetables daily.

In the context of the relationship between diet and cancer, it has been known for some time that people from the Mediterranean region are much less likely to develop prostate cancer than other Europeans. The reason for this would appear to be that their diets are rich in processed tomato products of the sort used in pizzas and pasta sauces. It is clear that only *cooked* tomatoes are protective, and the active ingredient that confers this protective effect would appear to be an agent called lycopene. Lycopene appears in tomatoes only as a result of cooking, the process changing the chemical nature of tomatoes.

Certainly, pursuing a diet of pizza and pasta would seem to be a most pleasant way of reducing the risk of developing prostate cancer. However, it is not clear how long you have to be on such a diet to increase your protection against getting prostate cancer. The Heinz Corporation, which buys up 80% of the world's production of tomatoes, was enormously interested in these observations, unique evidence of the military-industrial complex having a positive health benefit!

A number of studies have analysed the importance of trace elements such as zinc and selenium in the prevention of many cancers. The results would appear to suggest that there is a minor role for these elements in protecting against prostate cancer, but as yet it is unclear quite how significant this is. There is very little evidence that a normal diet is deficient in these trace elements, although some dietary pundits will comment that conventionally accepted standards are suboptimal assessments of requirements.

Conclusion

The evidence currently available suggests that the risk of future generations of men developing prostate cancer could possibly be reduced by a simple and healthy dietary management, so my advice to you is to eat more vegetables, pasta and pizza. However, it is very important to note that once a cancer has developed there is little objective evidence to support the view that changing diet will make the cancer go away or prolong survival. In fact, changing diets in these circumstances may even be detrimental, causing significant weight loss, affecting your life quality and jarring relationships by making your partner think that what she has fed you over the years has caused your cancer. If you do intend making drastic changes to your diet, I suggest you first discuss this with your doctor. Some of the organisations and support groups listed in Chapter 17 also offer dietary advice.

DIET : PREVENTION	
DO	**DON'T**
Eat at least five portions of fruit and vegetables a day.	Don't eat too much meat.
Enjoy eating pizza and pasta.	Drink excessive amounts of milk.
Avoid excessive smoked foods.	
Use soya products.	

CHAPTER THREE

The Journey to Diagnosis

The time taken to achieve a diagnosis of prostate cancer is longer than for any other tumour. A survey of practice in the United Kingdom published in 2000 showed that the average time between the patient presenting himself to his doctor with symptoms and receiving a diagnosis was ten weeks. In the current climate of blame and litigation, one might be tempted to think that the length of time taken would be the fault of the doctors involved with the care of the patients with this condition, but it is clearly not. As you will see, the reasons for this are many.

The Development of Symptoms

One of the most significant causes of delay is the non-specific nature of the symptoms of prostate cancer. The most common symptom is urinary frequency – that is, the increased need to pass urine. However, urinary frequency on its own is not diagnostic of cancer; the symptom is shared with benign enlargement of the prostate (BPH), which is a non-malignant condition and is virtually universal in older men.

Classically, urinary frequency will have developed gradually over many years, and because of the gradual nature of the change you may have adapted your lifestyle to fit in with your symptoms. Because urinary frequency is insidious in its onset and because it could be ascribed to BPH, you may view the symptom as unimportant until it becomes critical. Likewise, since the symptom is shared with benign enlargement of the prostate and malignancy is difficult to diagnose in general practice, the majority of patients will be referred on without an indication that the need for hospital review is in any way urgent.

There are other symptoms. Sometimes, when there is significant obstruction to the flow of urine from the enlarged prostate, the bladder may not empty completely. When the bladder is unable to empty completely, urine infections may become a problem. These infections are characterised by an increasing need to pass water, pain in the penis when passing water, a temperature and the feeling that the bladder has not emptied fully. This is called a *urinary tract infection* and should be assessed by examination of a specimen of urine in the microbiology department of the local hospital. Because urinary tract infections are very unusual in both men and women of middle or older age groups, they are almost always suggestive of a significant problem and require proper investigation.

It is unusual for a cancer of the prostate gland to cause any other symptoms unless the disease has spread from the prostate to involve other parts of the body. If there is spread, then the commonest symptom is pain in the bones. However, arthritic pains are very common, and so please don't think that your arthritis is due to cancer. Symptoms such as blood in the urine are extremely unusual but may occur in later stages of the illness.

The following chart shows you how to proceed if you develop symptoms.

Symptoms and what to do about them: patient's progress

Getting up more than twice
each night to urinate   Urine infection

Visit GP
Patient's story assessed.
Physical examination.
Blood tests, including those
for the kidneys and a PSA test.

Hospital referral to a urologist or oncologist

Further blood tests and X-rays

Review by the consultant with the results of tests

Raised PSA   Normal PSA, but
                                         significant symptoms

TRUS and biopsy
                                         TURP

Diagnosis and treatment

                                         Relief of symptoms in the
                                         majority of patients

Visiting Your Doctor

If you develop urinary symptoms, you should not be reticent about discussing your problems with your GP. Your doctor should assess your general physical condition and then, more specifically, examine you for bladder enlargement and any change in the prostate outline. Bladder enlargement is felt in the lower part of the tummy by pressing just above the pubic bone and can be confirmed by what is called percussion. This involves the tapping of the finger on the lower part of the tummy and hearing the different echoes that the tapping finger elicits from the abdominal contents. The sound of an enlarged bladder would be deeper than the sound of the echoes from the gas in the bowel. By this means, a diagnosis of enlargement of the bladder can be established.

The prostate shape can be examined only by a rectal assessment. If you have a suspected diagnosis of prostate enlargement, you will be asked to lie on your side on the doctor's couch and curl into a foetal position, drawing your legs up to your stomach. The doctor will place some lubricating jelly on a gloved finger and insert that finger through the anus. About 1^1/2 inches from the anus, the prostate can be felt. In normal configuration, its shape is like a walnut. With age, the walnut may become the shape of a plum, becoming bigger with benign enlargement of the prostate, and changing its shape to become knobbly if a tumour is present.

After the examination, if the doctor feels that there may be a problem with your prostate, he will carry out blood tests.

Some will be routine assessments of kidney function and a blood count, but more specifically the GP will measure levels of prostate specific antigen (PSA) within the blood stream. Because PSA is made by the normal prostate, blood levels can be elevated in normal men who do not have cancer but do have prostate enlargement. For this reason the normal range increases with age, and is up to 3.5 ng/l in 55-year-olds, 4.5 ng/l in 65-year-olds and 5.5 ng/l in 75-year-olds.

In the range of PSA values from above normal up to 10 ng/l, just 25% of men will have cancer. When PSA is up to 40 ng/l, just 40% of men will have cancer. In other words PSA is not a very good test for prostate cancer, a conclusion made even more substantial by the fact that a man can have a malignancy with a normal PSA result. A recent patient came to me to request a biopsy because his brother had the disease. His PSA result – at the age of 69 years – was 2.5 ng/l. The biopsy was positive.

If the symptoms are significant and your doctor's clinical suspicion is of cancer, a referral will be made to a hospital doctor. This referral should be to a consultant urologist, or to an oncologist if a diagnosis of cancer is suspected. The waiting time for such an appointment is subject to a government recommendation, which at the time of writing is two weeks. That is, a hospital consultant is currently required to review a patient with suspected prostate cancer in the outpatients department within two weeks of receipt of the letter of referral from the GP. The majority of patients with these symptoms will be found to have BPH and their care will remain in the hands of the urologist.

In the Outpatients Clinic

As an outpatient with suspected prostate cancer, you should expect to see a consultant at your first visit. Unfortunately, a lot of clinics are terribly oversubscribed and this may not be possible. Instead, you will be seen by a junior doctor who will confer with his consultant over your case. After a variable period of waiting, you will be called into the consulting room. There, a similar process to that experienced in your GP's surgery will take place. A history of your symptoms will be taken, an examination performed and blood tests arranged. Additional tests will also be organised.

Ultrasound examination

These tests should include a *transrectal ultrasound examination* (or TRUS) of your prostate. In this test a small cylindrical tube about the size of a finger will be inserted into your rectum. This is an ultrasound probe which emits high-frequency sound waves. These waves bounce back from the body's internal structures and produce a computerised image on a screen.

This image gives the radiologist an idea as to the outline of your prostate and the look of the internal structure of the gland. However, there is no correlation between this internal appearance and pathology – *pathology* means the appearance of this tissue when examined under the microscope – and for this reason further investigations need to be carried out.

In addition to providing information about the configuration of the prostate, the ultrasound probe gives an idea of the shape of the structures surrounding the prostate, such as the

33

seminal vesicles. It can also establish whether or not there are changes in the capsule of the prostate to suggest that the gland may have been breached by tumour.

Biopsy

The transrectal ultrasound examination (TRUS), is carried out in the department of radiology. The doctor ordering the investigation from clinic may also ask for biopsies – the removal of samples of tissue for examination – to be carried out at the same time. These biopsies are performed with the aid of small, spring-loaded needles in the ultrasound probe which are inserted into the prostate through the wall of the rectum. Six core biopsies are generally taken when using these needles. Because the needles are spring-loaded, their insertion is sudden and may cause some discomfort – many patients feel some pain, but a lot feel none whatsoever. The biopsy needles are withdrawn and the specimens put in pots for further examination. The whole procedure should take between 10 and 20 minutes to complete.

About 1–2% of patients develop an infection after the procedure. They run a temperature which may be high, and require treatment with antibiotics and sometimes hospitalisation. It is very common for there to be a little rectal bleeding but this should stop after a day and is very unlikely to be more than a few drops. Occasionally there may be a trace of blood in the urine but, again, this should stop after a day or so.

The specimens taken from your prostate are processed in the pathology department of the hospital. They require fixing so that the specimens can be processed by cutting and staining. This may take two to three days to complete, and is followed by an examination under the microscope of the material from the prostate gland. The pathologist – the doctor who examines this material – will then give an opinion as to the degree of infiltration of the prostate by tumour and the type of tumour that is present – a process known as 'staging' and 'grading' (*see* p.36, Prostate Cancer: Stage and Grade).

The tumour may be low grade, that is of relatively benign appearance, and involve only a small proportion of the cores of prostate obtained at TRUS. Alternatively, it may be high grade, that is very malignant, and involve all of the specimens. There is no real way of predicting the outcome of the biopsies from the rectal ultrasound. However, technologies constantly change and there is now some evidence that magnetic resonance imaging may be better than ultrasound for diagnostic purposes, but this is very much debated. There is also some hope that ultrasound techniques will also develop so that new contrast agents, given intravenously and travelling to the prostate, will give us clues as to what's going on in terms of pathological processes.

Once the ultrasound and blood tests have been carried out, if you have a suspected diagnosis of prostate cancer the next step is for your case to be reviewed in clinic. This review should take place within two weeks of the initial appointment.

Clinical Review and Further Investigations

In clinic, the doctor will review your PSA levels and the biopsy results together and assess the next step in your journey to treatment. This step will depend on whether the cancer is localised – that is, confined to the prostate gland – or has spread beyond it. Overall, in England and Wales about 60% of patients will have a cancer that has spread. This is a higher proportion of patients than in the USA. One of the reasons for this is likely to be that fewer UK men are screened than US males: only 1% as compared to 20%. It is thought that this may lead to the excessive diagnosis and treatment of indolent cancers in the USA – but the jury is still out about this.

To define the extent of spread of the cancer, the clinician will make a note of your symptoms and carry out an examination. The examination will be of the abdomen, lymph glands in the neck and of the prostate itself. The doctor will feel your tummy and assess whether or not the liver is enlarged or if there are abdominal glands that he is able to feel. He will prod around in your groin to see whether or not there are any enlarged glands that suggest the possibility of spread of the tumour. A rectal examination will also be performed. The clinician will assess with his finger the outline of your prostate and the possibility of involvement of surrounding structures. He is able to feel the outline of the seminal vesicles, which are the ducts that collect and retain sperm and prostatic fluid.

Prostate Cancer: Stage and Grade

Prostate cancer is described according to its extent within the gland and its microscopic appearance. The extent, that is the degree of spread, is known as the *stage*, whereas the microscopic appearance is described as the *grade*.

Staging

A universal system of staging is applied to all cancers and is synchronised by the World Health Organisation. This is called the TNM stage, where T defines the local stage of the tumour, N describes spread to lymph nodes, and M the presence of metastases. An attempt will be made to stage the prostate cancer from the clinician's examination. The clinical staging is as follows:

T	Primary Tumour
T0	No tumour palpable
T1	Tumour in one lobe of the prostate
T2	Tumour involving both prostate lobes
T3	Tumour infiltrating out of the prostate to involve seminal vesicles
T4	Extensive tumour, infiltrating local structures
N	**Nodal status**
N0	No nodes
N1	one-sided nodes
N2	Bilateral nodes
N3	Fixed regional nodes
N4	Juxta regional nodes
M	**Metastases**
M0	No metastases
M1	Metastases

You should be aware that staging definitions do change and there are further refinements of the tumour staging system.

PSA Levels and Staging

The clinician will also take great note of the PSA results, as PSA levels reflect the extent of spread of prostate cancer. If the results of the PSA levels are over 100 ng/ml then it is likely that the tumour is no longer confined to the prostate alone and that there will be spread of the disease to bones or lymph nodes. Levels between 20 and 100 are associated with spread beyond the prostate but not necessarily to bones or lymph nodes. Levels below this are associated with a much lower chance of spread.

Grading

The prostate cancer grading is a relative description of the appearance of the elements of the prostate under the microscope. Tumour that appears most closely related to normal prostatic tissue is described as *well differentiated*. Tumour that is least like the parent tissue is described as *poorly differentiated*, whilst tumour that is intermediate in appearance is described as being of *moderate* grade.

A further system of classification was established by Gleason, an American pathologist, who described prostate cancer as being of five grades, where grade 1 is the most like normal tissue and grade 5 the least like it. There is a further Gleason grading which is called the *Gleason combined grade*. In this, a summation is made of a Gleason score to 5, with two areas described: the most predominant pattern and the second most common pattern. A Gleason 3 + 3 score would indicate a tumour of moderate grade with very little variation, where-

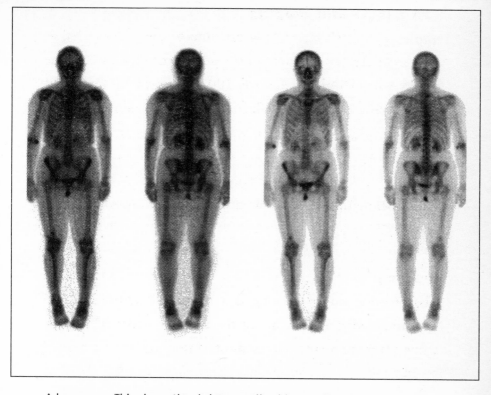

A bone scan. This shows the skeleton outlined by a radioactive chemical which has been injected into the bloodstream.

as a Gleason 1 + 5 score would indicate a tumour where there are elements of good and poor appearance. The significance of these scores relates to the prognosis of the tumour and is particularly important in the management of localised prostate cancer – that is, when the disease has not escaped from the prostate gland. A poorly differentiated cancer, that is a cancer of high Gleason grade, unfortunately has a poorer outlook than a well differentiated or low Gleason grade tumour.

39

Having completed the examination, the doctor will book further tests booked from clinic. These will include a bone scan to define whether or not the tumour has spread to involve the bones, and a CT scan or MR scan to assess your abdomen and pelvis.

Bone scan

The bone scan tests involve the injection of a radioactive tracer into a vein. The radiation dose is very small and will cause you no harmful effects. The tracer is taken up preferentially by blood vessels around bone and therefore helps to show whether or not the cancer has spread into the surrounding bone, which is where prostate cancer prefers to travel. Two to four hours after the injection of the tracer, images will be taken of your body. For this you will be required to lie on a bed in the radiology department. A Gamma camera, which is like a large X-ray machine in appearance, is then positioned over you and moves slowly from one end of your body to the other, collecting images of the emissions from the radioactive tracer.

Abnormalities in the uptake of the tracer are not specific to cancer, and may occur if you have degenerative disease of the spine or if you have fallen and bruised your ribs. The term 'degenerative disease of the spine' simply refers to changes to the spine resulting from the wear and tear that comes with old age. These changes are commonly seen in the lower spine, and may not be diagnostic of cancer. Similarly, minor trauma to the ribs can cause an increase in blood flow and therefore an increase in the take-up of the tracer, so isolated single changes within a rib are generally thought not to be diagnostic of the spread of cancer.

CT and MR scanning

Computerised tomography (CT) scanning is a complex process which involves a summation of digitised computer images of the soft tissues of the body. This is a complicated way of saying that many X-rays are taken of you and these are then added up by a computer in a way that allows us to see how you look inside. For a CT scan you will be required to lie on an X-ray table and have a series of X-rays taken of the internal contents of your abdomen and pelvis. This process takes approximately 15 minutes. The films are then reviewed by a radiologist and assessments made on the possibility of spread of the cancer. Prostate cancer may spread to lymph nodes, which are the internal glands within the abdomen and pelvis. If lymph nodes in the abdomen and pelvis are above 1cm in size, then there is a possibility of the spread of cancer to these nodes.

The results from studies which have compared the pathology of lymph nodes taken at operation to the images taken by CT scanning clearly show that there is no reliable correlation between lymph node size and the possibility of tumour involvement. In fact, there is a 60% error either way between lymph node enlargement and pathology. Lymph nodes may be enlarged on CT imaging but contain no tumour and vice versa.

CT scanning uses conventional X-rays, whereas magnetic resonance (MR) scanning involves the use of magnetic fields to obtain an image. The body's tissues are magnetised within an active magnetic field and an image obtained by measuring the speed of relaxation of the tissues after the field has been turned off. This is a complex process, as one might imagine from this brief description. The images obtained by MR scanning are similar in many ways to those obtained by CT, and the choice between the two to define the degree of spread of a cancer of the prostate depends really on the physician's preference for the images and the local availability of scanners.

As mentioned earlier, the purpose of all of these investigations is to define the degree of spread of a tumour. Defining the degree of spread allows your doctor to make a judgement as to treatment, which can then be discussed with you. These treatments will be explained in later chapters. First, however, it is important to understand the potential psychological and emotional effects of a diagnosis of prostate cancer. This is what we will look at in the next chapter.

THE JOURNEY TO DIAGNOSIS

Symptoms/PSA screening

↓

GP

↓

Urologist or oncologist

↓

Trus biopsies

↓

CT/MR scanning

+

Bone scanning

↓

Treatment

CHAPTER FOUR

The Diagnosis of Cancer

Cancer has earned itself a fearful reputation. In the past its diagnosis had a tendency to shatter lives and leave its victims feeling helpless and hopeless. But this popular view of cancer, which is still widely held in some sectors of the population, is now outdated. The treatment of cancer has evolved and generally speaking our attitude to the disease has changed. The issues of life quality now weigh strongly on the minds of the physicians who treat cancer. Drugs that ease pain are used with a liberality that was unheard of thirty years ago, and new medicines have been developed that effectively relieve most of the worst symptoms of cancer. Modern prostate cancer treatments are effective and are given with an increasingly significant chance for a positive response.

In these modern times a diagnosis of cancer no longer equates to a death sentence: a significant proportion of people with cancer are completely cured of their illness, whilst a further proportion may have their symptoms eased for a significant period of time. *Survival is a probability not a slim possibility.*

From my own experience, it is clear that many patients

accept their diagnosis, and do so with calmness. However, the circumstances in which they do so are not always facilitative of this. Patients are often told that they have cancer in an out-patient clinic setting. You may have waited for an hour and a half or longer in a crowded waiting area before being taken into a small consulting room. The doctor may well have seen forty patients already during that clinic. Although he will be doing his best, it is often difficult to give each patient the proper amount of time to explain and talk through the situation. Within what may seem like only a few minutes, you will have been given the diagnosis and offered a course of treatment.

In such circumstances it can be difficult to take in and deal with the information that you are given. Even if the out-patient environment is more conducive, you may be affected by psychological and/or emotional factors. When a patient is told that he or she has cancer, their immediate reaction is frequently one of absolute shock. In fact, in some patients this shock may be so profound that they are no longer able to hear what the doctor is saying to them. All they hear is their own thoughts echoing in their head. Generally speaking, these thoughts are of the most negative kind, such as 'I have got cancer, and I'm going to die'. Against such competition the rest of the doctor's words, however reassuring they may be, simply do not register.

With the shock that follows a diagnosis of cancer, the patient may have little memory of the details of their illness described by the clinician. The doctor's description of the illness may have been inaccurately heard or misinterpreted. It may even be remembered variably, with the patient repeating their description of events in different ways depending upon the person they are talking to.

For the above reasons it is important that patients who may receive a diagnosis of cancer are accompanied to the out-patients clinic by a friend or companion who can sit in on the consultation and who will be able to take them through the course of their illness. There are also a number of positive steps you can take. If in doubt, ask the doctor to repeat what he or she has said. If possible, make written notes of the conversation. This will give you something *concrete* to refer to once you have left the consulting room, rather than having your thoughts run amok with what the doctor *might have said*.

After the Diagnosis

The emotional reactions that follow a diagnosis of cancer take a course that can be defined in psychological terms. The initial shock is frequently followed by a period of *denial*. This denial can take many forms and be of varying degrees. It may be short-lived and evaporate in seconds or it may last many weeks. Characteristically, a patient in this state of denial will disbelieve the diagnosis. You may think that the diagnosis was wrong, that the biopsy results were inaccurate or that you have been given the result of another patient's diagnosis. In some patients, denial becomes the overwhelming factor in their lives. They may decide at a subconscious level that the mere thought of having cancer is so profoundly unbearable that they will carry on as normal. They may take themselves away from any medical intervention, deciding to discharge themselves from clinic, and will attempt to live a life that completely denies the diagnosis they have been given.

Denial can take many forms. For some patients the principal reason for denying the existence of their cancer is that they are unable to deal with the potential side-effects of treatment, especially the loss of libido associated with the diagnosis and treatment of prostate cancer. But this extreme reaction to the emotional stress of the diagnosis of prostate cancer is very unusual. For the vast majority of patients denial is quickly followed by the next step in the psychological process of coming to terms with the diagnosis of malignancy.

This next step is described as *guilt*. In this state the patient feels that the cancer has come as a punishment; therefore they are guilty, and so they must have done something wrong in their lives. They then examine their lives, looking for the causes of their punishment or for something to feel guilty about. They decide that they have got cancer because they were unfaithful to their wife in 1982, or because they have eaten too much meat, or simply because they have 'done something wrong'. However, punishment is *not* the reason for cancer.

In the 19th century it was commonly thought that tuberculosis was caused by depression, by dietary factors and by lifestyle. Patients with tuberculosis tried their best to change their diets and to eliminate the psychological causes of their illness, and so it is with cancer today. A remarkable medical scientist called Koch discovered the cause of tuberculosis – a bug called the TB bacillus. All the myths that related to the causes of tuberculosis disappeared. Everybody understood that their illness was caused by an infection, that it was nothing to do with their lifestyles. So it is with cancer today. There is no guilt associated with the diagnosis of cancer, and there is absolutely no need for you to feel guilty if you develop the disease. Cancer has come, and it is bad luck that it has happened. Feeling guilty about it is a self-imposed punishment that is best avoided.

When patients have moved through this phase of guilt most come to another stage in the process of acceptance of their condition. This stage is marked by a profound sense of *grief*, and is a period in which, quite understandably, there is a mourning for one's fate. The grief may be so intense that it disrupts family life. Often the grieving is not so much for the loss of self, but rather for the effects that loss of self may have upon one's family and friends. A father may grieve for the daughters and sons that he will leave behind and worry about how they will cope without him. A husband may grieve for the wife who will be left alone. He may wonder what she will do for companionship, how she will cope with the bills that he has always paid, how she will manage financially and how she will live without him. This period of grief can be totally overwhelming and it is, for many men, the hardest burden to bear.

In some cases the grief may also be for the dissolution of self that comes with death; for the loss of our senses – no more green fields to see, or voices of children to hear; for the loss of the comfort of everyday life, the good, the bad, the beautiful, even the nastiness. For some patients who mourn the possible loss of life, the smallest things can assume a most profound beauty. For these patients their grief gives way to a heightened sense of what it means to be really alive, in which their encounter with cancer becomes a life-enriching journey of self-discovery. And finally comes *acceptance*, acceptance of fate, and with that acceptance there is peace.

As a doctor, I marvel at the cheerfulness with which many of my patients greet their diagnoses. For the great majority, a diagnosis of cancer is not an unbearable burden. For many others, acceptance comes as they progress through all the stages of dealing with the diagnosis to an understanding of how they will deal with their disease. For some the diagnosis is, quite extraordinarily, a relief. Patients often tell me that they have been waiting with anxiety for this moment all their lives, and now that the diagnosis has come they are able to place their lives in context and can get on with living without fear, guilt or major constraint.

If you have received a diagnosis of cancer, there is always the possibility that you will run into an emotional sticking point somewhere along the line – whether it is guilt, grief, or mourning for lost opportunities or for the life you previously led. It is important that you pass through all the emotional stages of dealing with your disease. Getting stuck emotionally can add to any stress that may already have been triggered by your diagnosis. For this reason I would encourage you to talk the issues through with the people who care for you, wife, children, friends and professionals. Do not spare your family from discussion: they will find this lack of involvement distressing. Contrary to media representation, the medical profession is there to help in these matters. It may be helpful to talk through your situation with your doctor and to tell him of any worries you may have. Sometimes medication may be necessary to help you through, and antidepressants and medicines that help anxiety may be prescribed. There are a number of caring organisations and support groups that can also help, and details of these are provided for you in Additional Information at the back of this book.

THE DIAGNOSIS : EMOTIONAL STAGES

DENIAL

↓

GUILT

↓

GRIEF

↓

ACCEPTANCE

CHAPTER FIVE

Choosing Treatment

Following a positive diagnosis of cancer, the next step is to decide which is the most appropriate course of treatment for you. These are modern times. The days have long gone when patients were told what treatments they should have and the doctor's recommendations were followed unquestioningly. Nowadays, patients are better informed and medical practice is frequently questioned. With the apparent opening up of society has come the opportunity for patients to discuss the choice of treatments available to them. However, as the following story illustrates, this opportunity can bring with it an awful uncertainty.

On a ward round a few years ago I stopped to talk with a patient of whom I was particularly fond. She was a photographer and had breast cancer. She was unwell because her tumour had spread to her lungs and liver. I presented her with the options for her treatment. One option was a form of intravenous chemotherapy – 70% of all the patients treated with this treatment would have an improvement in their cancer – but unfortunately the disease would be likely to return. The side-effects of this particular treatment would include hair loss and vomiting, together with the risk of infection. I advised my patient that she could alternatively try a therapy that was less effective, having a chance of success in about 40% of patients. Treatment would again be given intravenously and was unlikely to cause any nausea or hair loss. Unfortunately, just as with the more toxic therapy, after a period of time the cancer would return.

My patient listened to the treatment options and at the end of our chat she asked me if she could think things over. I said that of course she could, and we carried on with our ward round, with Sister leading and Mark Bower, the House Officer, trailing behind. As we were leaving her bedside, the patient called Mark back. He sat on the edge of the bed and the two started to talk. Meanwhile, Sister and I carried on with our ward round. When Mark rejoined us a little while later, I asked him, 'What was that all about, then?' He replied, 'Well, she thinks that you have no idea as to what is the best treatment for her. And what's more she feels that if you don't know, how on earth could she be expected to make a judgement as to what's best for her?'

This was a remarkable experience for me. Remarkable because it seemed to show that an independent, highly educated women who is thoughtful and in touch with the modern world was made uneasy by the presentation of the available options and the fact that there was no one clear way in which her illness could be managed. At the risk of appearing terribly out of sync with modern perceptions, I must state that in this patient's case her disquiet about the possibility that there were options in the ways that her illness was managed made her feel insecure, and this insecurity was not particularly good for her.

Every so often my car needs servicing. It is then, with the greatest of pleasure, that I visit Graham Humphrey, my car doctor. "Humphrey" immediately puts me at ease by asking me: 'Have you been brilliant today?' I, of course, demur, but I know that he has been brilliant because every single car that ever visits his garage is cured. Humphrey then asks what the problem is with my car. When I tell him that it's the brakes, within a few moments the car is jacked up, the wheels are off and the brakes are inspected. He tells me it's the brake pads and adds, 'We'll soon fix that for you.' The car is then fixed. And so it has been for the many years that Humphrey has looked after my cars. There was the sixteen-year-old Mini and now there is a nine-year-old Renault. I can rely on Humphrey; he knows what to do. He fixes what's wrong with the car; it is better again.

When I go and see him about the brakes, I am not offered a choice of brake pads or brake shoes. I am not told that this or that brake shoe or pad will cost me this or that and last for such and such a time. I'm just given new brake pads or brake shoes, or whatever it is. It's sorted out for me, and I am left with my problem solved and no anxiety whatsoever about what I'm meant to do about my little car.

Of course, one can argue that human bodies are not like cars and that car brakes are not nearly as important as a potentially life-threatening illness. Sure, but one can also argue that, when the subject under discussion is human life rather than a car's brakes, it is even more important that the clinician appears confident, knowing exactly what to do and presenting the management of the patient's condition to him without the anxieties that are attendant on options. I do, of course, give an extreme example of the dichotomy that faces patients. But the reality is that patients must be properly informed about how to manage their condition.

There are many different ways in which prostate cancer can be managed, and this is because there is as yet no proof that there is *one* certain and 'correct' way to manage prostatic cancer. In medicine, certainty about treatment options is gathered from an analysis of the results of randomised clinical trials. This involves patients with the same condition being randomly allocated to one type of treatment or another and the relative advantages of the different treatments being compared. Proof of which treatment is best comes from an analysis of the results of such a trial.

In the case of localised prostate cancer, the treatment options include observation (where treatment is given if the patient develops symptoms), radiotherapy and radical surgery. Because these treatments have never been compared in a trial involving significant patient numbers, we have to rely on unreliable evidence – evidence that comes from single institutions where a comparison with other treatment forms has not been carried out. Observation without active treatment leads to an 87% chance of ten-year survival for patients with well and moderately differentiated tumours, and a 34% ten-year survival rate for patients with poorly differentiated tumours. Single institution studies suggest that there are similar results from radiotherapy or surgery for well differentiated cancer. For poorly differentiated tumours, however, surgeons argue that survival chances are greatly improved by radical surgery and range up to 77%. These figures are of questionable validity because it is argued that there is a significant bias in the selection of patients for surgery – of patients who proceed to radical surgery just 55% have organ-confined disease and are therefore potentially surgically curable. It is particularly relevant to note that surgery and radiotherapy have significant side-effects in terms of incontinence and impotence, whereas observation has no side-effects.

Because the case for one type of treatment as compared to another has not been proven in some areas of prostate cancer management, clinicians cannot always say with absolute certainty what the best approach might be. This can cause understandable anxiety in some patients. So, in prostate cancer as in many other cancers, I believe it is important to try to explain to the patient exactly what options there are. If the patient is unable to make up his mind, it is then appropriate for the clinician to help him to arrive at a decision.

The following chapters explain the various options for treatment, taking you step by step through each treatment process as well as describing any possible side-effects. For some patients the effect the latter may have on their quality of life is an important factor in their decision-making process.

Later on in the book I describe the stories of some typical, real patients and the choices that they had to face. It is hoped that in these stories you will come across echoes of your own situation, and, in the resolution or lack of resolution of particular problems, find some help in deciding which of the available options is the best one for you. If you need further help, turn to Chapter 16, Quesions to Ask Your Doctor.

CHAPTER SIX

Localised Prostate Cancer (1)

Observation and Delayed Treatment (Watchful Waiting)

By localised prostate cancer, doctors mean prostate cancer that is confined to the prostate gland. That is, the cancer has not spread to involve bones or internal organs such as the lymphatic system. The assessment of localised disease is dependent upon the accuracy of the scanning techniques and local examination described in Chapter 3. These determine whether or not the cancer remains within the confines of the prostate gland. The likelihood of spread is also reflected in increased levels of PSA: levels of 15 or greater indicate a probability of spread of prostate cancer microscopically beyond the prostate.

The Management Options for Localised Prostate Cancer

There are three different ways of managing localised prostate cancer. These are:

- observation, with delayed treatment (also known as 'watchful waiting')
- radiotherapy, which includes brachytherapy
- surgery

It has to be said that opinions are divided on how best to manage localised prostate cancer. This lack of consensus is due to the fact that there has as yet been no major comparative trial to establish which of the treatment options is best for the patient with localised disease. One of the reasons for the lack of such a comparative trial is that surgeons appear to be convinced that surgery is the only way forward, curing all the patients that need to be cured, while many radiotherapists have similar views about the efficacy of radiation therapy.

There have been trials, however, of individual treatments and their efficacy. So we do know how successful radiotherapy is as a single treatment but not as a comparative treatment for localised prostate cancer. Similarly, we have results from single centres with regard to the effects of surgery in controlling prostate cancer. We also have some information about the way in which prostate cancer can be managed by delayed therapy. Unfortunately, in the absence of head to head comparisons of these three management techniques involving significant numbers of patients, the problem for the patient is to choose between the approaches. However, some patients turn this potential problem to their advantage by gathering as much information as possible that is relevant to their own particular case. For different approaches suit different patients, depending upon the type of disease they have, their age and the way they wish to lead their lives.

Observation and Delayed Treatment (Watchful Waiting)

For many patients, prostate cancer is a relatively indolent disease – a cancer that causes no significant problems in their lives. For a disease that causes no problems, it seems sensible to pursue a course of action where no treatment is given. The major reason that no treatment is a consideration for some patients is that no treatment – otherwise known as 'watchful waiting' – has no side-effects, whereas both surgery and radiotherapy certainly do cause significant problems.

The 'watchful waiting' approach has been subjected to an analysis in 828 men with prostate cancer. In this analysis the patients were brought together from a number of different trial results and an overview was derived. All of these patients were observed, and hormonal therapy was given when there was evidence of symptomatic progression of their cancer. For those patients with well or moderately differentiated cancers – i.e. cancers that appear to be least malignant under the microscope – 87% survived at ten years. This means that only 13% of these patients died as a result of prostate cancer. For those patients with poorly differentiated tumours – i.e. those that appear the most malignant under the microscope – survival fell to 34% at ten years.

These results appear to be of great significance for patients with prostate cancer confined to the prostate. They suggest that there is an excellent prospect of survival without any treatment, and this is very important when one considers that the average age at diagnosis of prostate cancer is 72. If a man of

72 has an 87% chance of surviving 10 years without any treatment of his prostate cancer, this is a chance that this patient may consider it reasonable to take. However, for the patient with a poorly differentiated cancer, the decision for active treatment may be a better option. These options are discussed in later chapters. Survival figures need to be considered in the context of the average life expectancy for a man, which is 74.9 years in the UK.

It has been argued that delaying treatment until symptoms indicate the need for intervention may be harmful to the patient with prostate cancer. The Medical Research Council in the UK organised a study in which patients with asymptomatic prostate cancer were either allocated to receive active treatment upon diagnosis or treatment was delayed until they became symptomatic. Nearly 800 patients were randomised into this study. Some of these had localised disease and some had cancer that had spread. The launch of the study caused a tremendous amount of negative publicity, with a number of major newspapers running campaigns which criticised the doctors carrying out the study. In their view, patients with cancer were not being treated and this seemed, to the journalists, to be anathema.

The results of this study, which was started in the mid-1980s and completed in the 1990s, showed that there was an increased risk of patients dying from prostate cancer and of suffering from significant complications of their disease if they were not treated early. However, it also appeared that these deaths and complications were mostly confined to those patients who had cancer that had spread from the prostate gland. In other words, those patients with disease confined to the prostate had no such risk. The study has clearly shown that, provided patients are relatively carefully monitored, watchful waiting for cancer of good microscopic appearance that is confined to the prostate gland is a safe option.

So we can conclude from this study that where the tumour is confined to the prostate gland and is of good appearance under the microscope delaying active treatment for prostate cancer is a suitable option. Much prostate cancer in this form will cause no problems for the person diagnosed and living with the disease. This option may also be a safe thing to do for patients with cancer that looks a little bit more aggressive under the microscope.

Prostate cancer, in its indolent form, has become increasingly diagnosed as a result of the successes of screening, particularly in Europe and the USA. With this increase, more and more patients will be faced with the dilemma of whether or not to be treated. This dilemma is easy to understand, for it can be difficult to come to terms with the fact that a cancer is present but doesn't need treatment. And yet this is the case for patients who have tumours of very good prognosis, tumours that will not impact upon their lives. For the majority of these patients, the steady approach of observation without active therapy until symptoms dictate would seem to be the most suitable option.

The following are my views on selection for the 'watchful waiting' option for patients with localised prostate cancer:

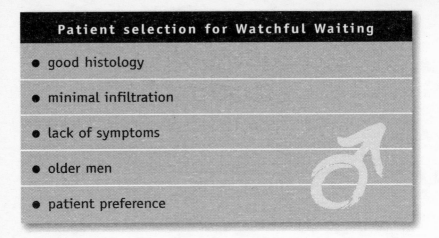

Patient selection for Watchful Waiting

- good histology

- minimal infiltration

- lack of symptoms

- older men

- patient preference

CHAPTER SEVEN

Localised Prostate Cancer (2)

External Beam Radiotherapy

In this chapter we look step by step at the second treatment option for localised prostate cancer: radiotherapy, which is a complicated process involving sophisticated machinery and highly trained medical and paramedical staff.

Planning

The first step in radiotherapy is termed *planning* – a word that precisely identifies the process. Radiotherapy planning involves the determination of the area within the body that requires treatment and the calculation of the radiotherapy dosage that is to be applied to the treatment area.

In the last decades of the 20th century, the planning process for prostate cancer was relatively unsophisticated. The patient would be catheterised and radio-opaque dye injected through the catheter into the bladder. The dye would show an outline of the bladder and the position of the catheter. This image would be shown on an X-ray of the patient, and the X-ray would be used in the planning process because the dye gives an impression of the position of the prostate gland, situated as it is at the base of the bladder. This X-ray would give the clinicians and radiographers an idea as to the position of the prostate within the body.

Scanning

In the 1990s and 2000s, modern centres have begun to use a CT scanner to identify the position of the prostate – computerised information is taken from the CT scanner and used directly to work out the precise position of the prostate. As can be imagined, this is a much more accurate process than using simple X-rays. An ordinary X-ray allows one to see internal solid structures, such as the bones, but it gives a very poor view of soft tissues, such as the bowel or the prostate. By contrast, CT scanning gives an excellent view of soft tissues. Computerised imaging also allows the precise identification of other internal organs, such as the rectum. This helps considerably in reducing the radiation dosages to normal tissues, such as the rectum, and allows the radiotherapy to be given more precisely to the prostate itself.

You may be asked to take a strong laxative dosage the night before and then be given a small enema on the morning of the CT scan. The radio-opaque dye in the enema will help outline the position of the bowel relative to the prostate. For the majority of CT scans additional contrast is required. Contrast material may be taken by mouth some hours before the scan or may be injected into your veins during the scan itself. This delineates and outlines the structures of the organs adjacent to the prostate. It may also outline the position of the bowel, arteries and veins, thus allowing a clearer image of the prostate to be obtained.

The scanning process itself is relatively straightforward. The machinery used looks like any other X-ray machinery and the process of having a scan causes no bizarre sensation. You are asked to lie on a hard table, and the scanner head is positioned just over the relevant area of the body. The scanning staff, who are called *radiographers*, then leave the scanning room and enter an observation area, which is partitioned from the scanner by a glass screen. Over a period of ten to fifteen minutes, CT scanning pictures are taken. Each image is taken in less than a second, after which the scanner head is automatically adjusted to take a picture in the next position.

Treatment Planning

The information obtained through scanning is sent from the CT computer to the planning computer in the radiotherapy department. Through the use of the planning computer, which is an expensive piece of machinery, images of the prostate are constructed. Radiotherapy dosages are calculated around these images. This complex and highly skilled process is carried out by physicists who calculate from the radiotherapy machines the dosage required to treat the prostate to a plan. The mathematical formulae that are used in planning take into account the effects of radiation on normal tissues and on malignant tissues. Radiotherapy beam dosages are calculated, and a plan is made as to the specifics of the administration of treatment.

Old-fashioned treatment, planned without the aid of computers, aims to deliver radiation in a treatment dosage with the outline of a small brick. This pelvic-brick treatment shape is likely to be delivered from two different points, one from the front of the body and the other from behind. However, the prostate is not shaped like a brick. In normal life it is shaped like a walnut and in malignancy it may have an irregular outline. Radiotherapy planning using computer technologies allows the delivery of radiation aimed around the shape of the prostate and usually from four different angles to the body. This technique is called *conformal radiotherapy*. The administration of radiation from various angles relative to the prostate gland limits the radiation dose to normal tissue. There is a further refinement of computerised planning which is called *intensity modulated radiotherapy*. This involves the application of relatively complex physics to step up the local dose of radiotherapy to the prostate whilst limiting the dosages to normal tissue.

Personnel

The amount of time required in planning the delivery of radiotherapy to the prostate is about three to four hours. Effective planning requires the combined skills of radiotherapists, physicists and radiographers, all of whom contribute to the prescription of radiotherapy treatment to the patient with prostate cancer. As a result of the deliberations of the team, a plan for radiotherapy treatment evolves. This plan is based upon the radiotherapy prescription – i.e. the dosage required to treat the prostate – and the geography of the prostate gland within the patient. Treatment dosage may be modified by the clinicians' views as to the patient's susceptibility to the effects of radiotherapy.

Simulation

The next step in the radiotherapy treatment process is called *simulation*, which is a dummy run for the real treatment. If you are to receive radiotherapy, you will be asked to come along to the radiotherapy treatment centre where you will be taken into the simulator room. This contains equipment just like an X-ray machine, but with a tremendous amount of accessory computer-based technology.

In the simulator room you will be asked to lie on the X-ray machine couch. Here the plan devised by the radiotherapy team will be applied to you, and the practicalities as to whether or not the treatment plan is appropriate and the delivery techniques accurate will be worked out. When the radiotherapy team is satisfied that their treatment plan is accurate, a small permanent tattoo mark will be made on your skin. This tattoo mark will be used to determine the positions of the radiotherapy delivery during the treatment process.

Treatment

If you are worried about the process of treatment with radiotherapy, this is entirely normal. After all, for anyone other than a cancer doctor or radiographer, it probably feels as though you are journeying into the black heart of darkness. One of the porters who worked in our department would explain to worried patients that they really had nothing to worry about. He would cheerfully and patiently explain that the radiotherapy process involved no pain, no heat, no electric shocks, no torture and was without any obvious immediate effect. His kind words were rightfully reassuring.

The appointment for radiotherapy treatment may follow some days after planning and simulation. In many centres there is a waiting list for radiotherapy, with the aim being to start treatment some six weeks from the diagnosis of prostate cancer. This may seem like a terrible delay. It is, in its emotional effects. Many patients feel that it is bad enough to have cancer but to wait for six weeks to start treatment is an additional intolerable burden. However, whilst it is clearly far from ideal because of the anxiety caused by the wait, there is in fact no good evidence to suggest that this lag period is harmful and leads to any chance for the cancer to spread.

What happens during radiotherapy

The machinery used to administer radiotherapy treatment looks just like a CT scanner or plain X-ray machine. Radiotherapy treatment machines are situated in hospital basements. The reason for this is that they contain radioactive sources. These sources are sealed to minimise environmental radiation leak. The basement rooms where they are located are surrounded by many metres of high density barium concrete, designed to damp down any radioactivity which, should there be an accident, which could be lethal to the hospital community of doctors, patients and paramedics, as well as to the general public in the area surrounding the hospital.

It is ironic to note that, because of the protection around the radiation source, the safest place to be in a nuclear war is the radiotherapy department of your local hospital!

So what is having radiotherapy like? Well, it starts with a descent into the hospital basement, and this descent for treatment may strike you as rather creepy – creepy because of the absence of windows, the artificial light and the strangeness of the medical environment. The smell, sights and sounds are all extraordinary and attempts are made to improve the strange atmosphere by making the setting a little more friendly. These attempts, which usually consist of plastic plants and pine cladding, very rarely work, frequently compounding the environmental alienation. It is only by going through the treatment process that you will get used to the bizarreness of it all.

The day you attend hospital for treatment is known as the 'first treatment day'. You will be asked to wait in a waiting area with other patients. This is a very good opportunity for you to meet other patients and talk with them about what to expect. There is nothing like the reassurance of a fellow patient that the whole process is not too bad to calm the nervous first timer. You need to remember that not all treatments are the same, or involve the same areas, so that other patients' experiences may not mirror your own.

When it is your turn for treatment you will called down to the basement of the department and taken into the radiotherapy treatment room by a radiographer, who will position you on the treatment couch. The radiographer will then orientate the treatment head of the radiotherapy machine in the correct position using laser beams to align the head of the machine with the tattoo that was applied to your body in the simulation room. The laser beams and the low light environment are rather like a bizarre, soundless discotheque. It's all very weird to those not used to hospital environments.

The radiographer will ask you to keep as still as you possibly can, and then he or she will leave the treatment room. This minimises his or her exposure to radiation. The staff will observe you from the machine control, using a video camera set up in the treatment room. After a few moments the radiotherapy treatment is given. The radiation, which takes the form of energy waves, will leave no external physical impression upon you. You will not even notice that it has been given. After less than a minute you will be allowed to get up from the treatment couch and leave the hospital.

In most centres the time taken from your arrival at the radiotherapy treatment centre to completion of your treatment will be in the order of 30–45 minutes. The whole process is really very straightforward once the complexities of planning and simulation have been completed.

The most common treatment plans involve daily treatment, apart from weekends, for a period of six weeks. In some centres treatment is given to higher dosages, and this may require either multiple daily attendances or a more protracted treatment course. The majority of people continue a normal life throughout their treatment, and most of the patients that I have referred for radiotherapy continue their normal daily routines around the period of the hospital visit. Many people continue to go to work daily.

Possible Side-effects

The process of radiotherapy treatment can be very tiring because of the physical effort of visiting hospital every day. There is additional fatigue that has its source its the emotional strain of having therapy, and this effect should not be under-estimated – emotions can also be tiring.

This tiredness tends to be cumulative and, towards the end of treatment, can be such that it is best to go with the flow and take time out to sleep during the day. Some people feel that the actual process of radiotherapy causes tiredness through a physical effect which is scientifically unexplained but real.

Cystitis and urethritis

About four weeks into treatment some people develop some side-effects from radiotherapy. The most common of these is due to the effects of radiotherapy on normal tissue, such as the urethra, which passes through the centre of the prostate. Radiotherapy to the urethra can cause some irritation – *urethritis* means inflammation of the urethra. As a result, cystitis-like symptoms may develop. That is to say, you may experience an increased need to urinate and some discomfort on urination. These symptoms are very common, usually increasing over the last two weeks of treatment and tending to recover one to two weeks after the completion of radiotherapy.

The symptoms are very variable in their intensity, ranging from little or no discomfort to a feeling comparable to needles pricking the inside of the penis during urination. There is little that can be done to make these symptoms better. Cranberry juice is often recommended but rarely proves to be of use. Patent medical cures such as Mist Pot Cit should be avoided at all cost because the potassium in these supplements can cause severe cardiac problems. Mist Pot Cit is a liquid medicine containing a chemical – potassium citrate – which is excreted into the urine. This process acidifies the urine and by this means relieves symptoms.

Proctitis

The other organ that is affected by radiotherapy is the rectum, and the timing of these effects is very similar to that of the effects on the urethra. The rectum is situated just behind the prostate and appears to be, glancing over the gland. There is always some radiation dose given to the rectum during prostatic radiotherapy. This radiation will cause irritation, just as it does in the urethra – *proctitis* means irritation or inflammation of the rectum. This irritation will lead to diarrhoea, the amount and frequency of which varies enormously from one patient to the next.

The diarrhoea can be treated, and treated successfully. The recommendation is to use drugs such as Lomotil or Codeine to slow down the passage of stools through the bowel. The diarrhoea should cease some two weeks after the completion of radiotherapy. Unfortunately, in some patients the radiation damage is such that permanent scarring results. This may lead to diarrhoea that doesn't go away, and sometimes rectal bleeding. In severe cases steroid enemas or even surgery are required for the condition.

Impotence

The other major side-effect of radiation therapy is on the patient's sex life. Generally, these effects are slow to kick in and may take several years to be noticed. This major problem is caused by radiation damage to the blood vessels which supply the nerves that control sexual function. This damage can be such as to make it impossible to have an erection. This is important, and it is common, so don't be shy about discussing it with your doctor.

It is estimated that up to 70% of men who have had normal sexual function become impotent as a result of radiotherapy. However, the effects of radiotherapy on potency can be relieved by a number of artificial means. Probably the easiest treatment for potency loss is Sidenafil, which is popularly known as Viagra. Taken just before intercourse, these tablets will allow about 40% of men to achieve an erection. Other, less acceptable methods, which are of less subtlety and interfere more with the loving process of sex, are vacuum pumps and internal mechanical prostheses. However, these devices should be tried should the easy approach of taking tablets fail. These devices are discussed in more detail in Chapter 9. It is very important to deal with this situation as early as possible and not ignore it. The earlier that Viagra, or more modern alternatives are tried, the more likely they are to work – and the later, the less likely.

Adjuvant Hormone Treatment

Additional treatment may be offered you. Patients may be given the choice of having extra treatment with hormonal therapy using therapies designed to suppress the male hormone. I discuss details of such treatment in a later chapter. It has been shown that these treatments decrease the risk of the cancer coming back in the prostatic area after radiotherapy. Only one study, amongst many, has shown an increase in life expetancy with this additional treatment. The downside is hot flushes and impotence, but these recover. No one knows what the correct period of time is that this extra treatment should be given.

Results

Patients who are selected for radiotherapy tend either to have elected for treatment on the basis that they do not want to have surgery, or because they are considered not to be fit enough medically for surgery. This means that the results of treatment with radiotherapy tend to be skewed by patient selection so that there are poorer results than with surgery. This is particularly the case for cancers of high Gleason grade, where just 15–30% of patients survive ten years. Much better results are seen with intermediate and low grade tumours, where survival rates may be similar to those seen for surgery – and indeed for observation and delayed therapy – with up to 80% surviving ten years or longer.

The following are my views on patient selection for the

external beam radiotherapy treatment option for patients with localised prostate cancer:

Patient selection for External Beam Radiotherapy

- patient preference

- well differentiated cancer – i.e. low Gleason grade

- small volume tumours

- potency not at issue

- age over seventy years

- any pre-existing history of colitis is a contra-indication to treatment, as colitis can be made worse

CHAPTER EIGHT

Localised Prostate Cancer (3)

Brachytherapy

Brachytherapy is the treatment of prostate cancer by the implantation of radioactive material into the prostate. Interstitial brachytherapy, to give it its full name, is increasingly popular. I am not sure why this should be the case, but it would appear that patients have the idea that this technique is futuristic and thus offers them an improved chance of success. But brachytherapy has been around for decades. As with the other options for prostate cancer treatment, the relative effectiveness of brachytherapy is difficult to evaluate because of the lack of a randomised controlled clinical trial comparing the results of brachytherapy treatment with standard radiation treatment, surgery or delayed therapy.

Patient Selection

The selection of patients for brachytherapy is defined by relatively strict criteria. Patients are excluded if:

- their Gleason grade is higher than 6
- their PSA levels are higher than 10 ng/ml
- their clinical stage is higher than T2a

These highly selected patients would also be likely to have a very good prospect for cure by standard radiotherapy or surgery, or indeed a very low chance of progression of their tumour without active treatment.

The Procedure

The delivery of interstitial brachytherapy is complex. After an initial assessment to ensure that you fulfil the entry criteria for inclusion in brachytherapy treatment, you will usually be admitted to hospital for your first assessment. This may be as a day case.

Assessment
After a preliminary assessment to ensure that you are fit for the anaesthetic procedure, you will be anaesthetised, an ultrasound probe will be inserted into your rectum and multiple measurements will be taken to assess the dimensions and configuration of the prostate and its relationship to other structures, such as the urethra. This procedure requires a relatively short anaesthetic, after which you return to the anaesthetic recovery room and, after a few hours, you will usually be discharged home.

Planning
The information that is obtained at the assessment provides the radiotherapists and planning physicists with the necessary details that help them to establish a treatment plan. Interstitial brachytherapy requires the insertion of radioactive seeds of iodine or palladium into the prostate. The positioning of these

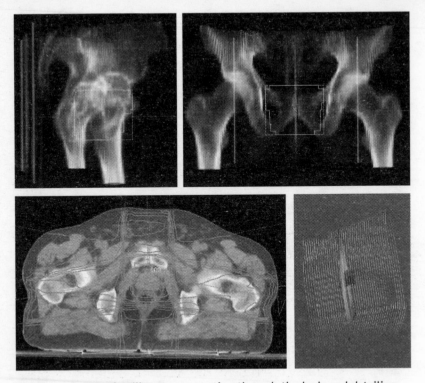

Theses are images detailing a cross section through the body and detailing radiotherapy dosage maps.

seeds is worked out from a knowledge of the geography of the prostate in each patient and from an understanding of the radiation emission characteristics of the implanted seeds. Radiotherapy is emitted from the seeds in a dosage that diminishes as the distance from the seeds increases.

The planning physicists work out the dosage distribution so that all areas of the prostate are treated with an adequate dosage of radiation and that no areas of the prostate are left out. Within this plan, the physicist has to be careful to make sure that dosages of radiotherapy delivered to the urethra are not excessive. If the dosage to the urethra is too high, complications could ensue. The process of planning interstitial brachytherapy for prostate cancer may take up to three hours.

Treatment

Once the plan has been created and further theatre time allocated, the radioactive pellets will be ordered and delivery organised. It is usual for patients who are to receive brachytherapy to have their second admission approximately two weeks from the initial planning session.

This second procedure is far more complicated than the first. The procedure requires an anaesthetic and an ultrasound probe inserted into the rectum. A metal grid is set up and secured to the operating table. Needles containing removable cores are insert-ed through the grid and then through the skin of the perineum – the area between the scrotum and the rectum – into the prostate gland. The depth of insertion of the needles determines the place-ment of the radioactive implants. The positioning of the needle tips is checked using the ultrasound probe and may be confirmed by the use of a conventional X-ray.

When the positioning of the needles is satisfactory and matches the defined radiotherapy treatment plan, the needles may be linked up through plastic tubing to an afterload delivery system – a machine that remotely and automatically posts the radioactive pellets to the prostate gland. The use of this machines limits radiation dosage to the doctors and nurses treating the patient, as the pellets supplied can be safely administered from a distance.

Alternatively, the radioactive pellets can be picked up with forceps and, with care, each pellet inserted through the hollow needles into the prostate, where they are left. This can be done without danger to the radiotherapist provided the pellets are kept at a reasonable distance from his hands and away from his body.

A typical brachytherapy treatment involves the insertion of up to forty pellets of iodine or palladium. The time taken for this procedure ranges from one and a half to three hours, depending upon the experience of the team. You are then returned to the anaesthetic recovery room, and from there to your ward. In the ward there will be no restriction on visiting – because the radiation emitted by the pellets only travels a short distance there is no significant radiation risk to your visitors.

Topping-up brachytherapy

Many patients think that brachytherapy has a significant advantage over external beam radiotherapy because the procedure is over and done with in a relatively short period of time. Although this may be the case for the brachytherapy itself, for many patients external beam radiotherapy is required in addition to the brachytherapy. This is because the brachytherapy alone will not necessarily deliver an effective treatment dose to the prostate, and so a top-up is required using conventional radiotherapy delivery systems and techniques.

Possible Side-effects

Immediate complications

After the procedure the patient will have some significant bruising to the perineum. This is perfectly understandable when you consider that up to forty needles may have been inserted through the perineum. Some engorgement of the prostate may occur, in which case you may experience some difficulty in urinating after the procedure. In many cases a urinary catheter will have been inserted into the prostate at the time of procedure and will be removed a day or so later. Occasionally patients will have bleeding from the prostate into urine, which tends to stop after a day or so. Rarely, infections causing temperatures and requiring antibiotic treatment may also happen.

It is frequently the case that a patient will also suffer some side-effects from the anaesthetic. These are generally very mild and include some tiredness or nausea. However, with modern anaesthetic techniques and anaesthetic agents, there is very little ill effect from anaesthesia and most people feel completely well afterwards.

The most common symptoms after brachytherapy are described as 'irritative'. Patients rush to go to the lavatory, urinate more frequently, and have a burning feeling in the urethra. These symptoms occur in up to a third of patients, generally last for a few weeks and, in most patients, resolve themselves. Rarely, symptoms may persist for several months. These urinary symptoms may become profound, and very occasionally incontinence is reported. It is rare, however, that the incontinence lasts beyond six months.

Proctitis

Radiation delivery to the prostate may also affect the rectum. If this occurs, patients may develop proctitis – irritation or inflammation of the rectum. The symptoms of proctitis are the frequent need to pass a motion, the feeling that a motion is present in the rectum and sometimes the passage of blood and mucus. Just like urinary symptoms, proctitis generally persists for a few weeks and usually resolves itself, rarely persisting beyond three to six months.

Impotence

As with external beam radiotherapy, brachytherapy can have a major impact on a patient's sex life. Those patients who had an active sex life prior to treatment may have difficulty in achieving or sustaining an erection. Erectile dysfunction, or impotence, unfortunately results in an inability to have intercourse, although the patient's libido – his sex drive – remains normal. This symptom is said to occur in up to 20% of patients. However, not all doctors are convinced that this figure is accurate. Radiotherapy causes damage to small blood vessels, known as *endarteritis*. The effects of this damage occur gradually, over a long period of time. It is thought that patients are more likely to retain sexual function if they are under the age of 50 at treatment than if they are older. In my view it is likely that impotence will be seen in an increasing number of patients as time goes by.

Results

There is only limited research study into the long-term results of the effects of brachytherapy on prostate cancer control. In one trial of patients who received Iodine[125]-based brachytherapy with or without additional external beam radiation therapy, results were reported after a median of ten years from treatment. During this period, just three of the 152 patients had died of prostate cancer, whilst 97 (64%) remained biochemically free of disease, with PSA values in the normal range.

The authors of this study comment on the rate of change of PSA levels. In brachytherapy, patients' PSA levels continue to fall very slowly, taking up to five years from treatment to reach their lowest point. This is in contrast with the expectation for conventional radiotherapy where levels should reach their low point at three to six months from the completion of treatment.

In summary, brachytherapy offers a very effective treatment for prostate cancer. However, I end with the caveat that has become something of a cliché in medicine, that this advantage needs to be confirmed by a clinical trial in which brachytherapy is compared with the more conventional approaches.

The following are my views on patient selection for the brachytherapy treatment option for patients with localised prostate cancer:

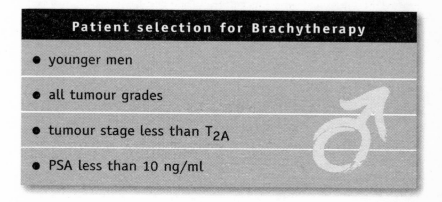

Patient selection for Brachytherapy

- younger men
- all tumour grades
- tumour stage less than T_{2A}
- PSA less than 10 ng/ml

CHAPTER NINE

Localised Prostate Cancer (4)

Radical Surgery

The aim of radical surgery for prostate cancer is to cure the patient by cutting out all tumour. Surgery for prostate cancer is major surgery. As such it may have major side-effects and carries with it the potential risks associated with all major surgery. It is also an operation that requires enormous skill – a skill that is refined with practice. A patient who is to undergo radical prostatectomy should be operated upon by a surgeon who has considerable experience of this technique, because the rate of complications decreases and the success of surgery increases with the experience of the surgeon. Ask your surgeon how many cases a year he does and you'll get a feel for his experience. And ask your GP if he would choose to be operated on by the surgeon he has referred you to.

Patient Selection

Patient selection for prostate cancer surgery is strict and only specific groups of patients are deemed operable. The reason for this is that the potential side-effects of surgery increase unless

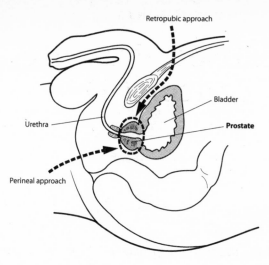

Surgical approaches to prostectomy.

very strict criteria are used to define a patient's operability. Those considered to be unsuitable for surgery are:

- patients older than seventy, because the side-effects are considered to be too great in this age group: wound healing may be delayed and mortality rates increase
- patients who have PSA levels of 15 or over, because these patients have a greater likelihood of spread of the prostate cancer beyond the confines of the gland and/or into neighbouring lymph nodes, therefore the operation is unlikely to be successful as it cannot be carried out with curative intent. Some surgeons will not operate on patients with PSA levels of 10 or over.
- patients who have existing medical conditions, such as heart failure or chronic lung diseases, because the consequences of the anaesthetic and of the surgery itself may be too great for them to survive the operation
- generally, but not always, previous radiotherapy

Those men who are under seventy years of age, have low PSA levels, no pre-existing significant medical conditions, and who, with informed consent, have agreed to the procedure, are considered to be suitable for radical prostatectomy. It is argued by sceptics that the selection criteria for surgery are so rigorous that only those patients with relatively mild forms of the disease and the best chance of cure are considered for operation.

The Run Up to Surgery

Radical prostatectomy has advanced as a surgical technique over the last twenty years due to the definition of the nerve supply to vital organs around the prostate. The nerves which pass around and through the prostate control sexual function, and so damage to them could lead to impotence. The operation has been refined so that damage to these vitally important nerves is limited. These improvements in technique have also meant that the side-effects of surgery may be less than before. The name of the operation has been changed to reflect these advances and is now called a *radical nerve-sparing prostatectomy*.

Prior to surgery, the patient with prostate cancer requires staging. That is, testing by scanning to find out whether the tumour has spread. The first of these scans is likely to be a rectal ultrasound – just as an ultrasound examination can be used to look at a baby in the womb, so it can also be used to examine the appearances of the prostate. The images produced show the general appearance of the prostate and whether or not the prostate capsule is penetrated by the tumour. It should be repeated at this point that the ultrasound results do not correlate with pathology. In other words, if the prostate were to be removed and examined microscopically by a pathologist, in the vast majority of patients no link would be found between the position of the tumour and the ultrasound appearance of the prostate.

A bone scan should be performed and a CT or MR scan of your abdomen and pelvis will be carried out.

The Operation

Admission to hospital is usually on the day before the operation. You will be booked in by a junior doctor and blood tests arranged. On the day prior to surgery, an anaesthetist will examine you, reviewing your overall medical state – in particular the state of your heart and lungs – to determine your fitness to undergo the procedure.

On the day of the operation you will be given a pre-med prior to surgery. This is an injection given several hours before the operation. The drugs that are administered in the pre-med help you relax and dry up lung secretions so that anaesthetic complications are reduced. After the injection your throat will feel very dry and you will become sleepy. You will be given a suppository which will cause the bowel to empty, making surgery easier and reducing the risks of side-effects, such as infection. You will also be fitted with thigh length anti-thromboembolism support stockings to prevent clots forming in your leg veins. Patients are usually given an injection of Heparin, a drug that prevents blood clots forming, under the skin. Blood clots form more commonly in people who have operations than in those who don't. An antibiotic may also be given.

Next you are wheeled to an anteroom outside the operating theatre. An anaesthetist will give you an injection into a vein, and within a few seconds you will be unconscious.

The surgical incision is usually abdominal. Rarely, it may be in the area of the perineum, which extends from the scrotum back to the anus. The surgeon will initially remove the iliac lymph nodes that drain lymphatic secretions from the prostate. Using a technique known as frozen section, the pathologist who is on standby waiting for the nodes to arrive from the operating theatre will examine these lymph nodes while the surgeon waits to proceed with the next operative steps. If there is any lymph node involvement, the operation will not continue. This is because lymph node involvement suggests further distant spread of the cancer, in which case an operation on the primary tumour would clearly be inappropriate. The operation proceeds if the pathologist finds no cancer cells in the lymph nodes.

The next step is for the surgeon to dissect down to the prostate. The urethra, which is the tube that conveys urine from the bladder through the penis, will be exposed and divided to reveal the rectum. The nerves that control erection lie between the prostate and the rectum. These are identified in the nerve-sparing procedure and not cut because cutting them will lead to complete loss of potency. At this point the prostate is exposed, together with the seminal vesicles – a system of tubes and ducts that contain semen and contract during ejaculation.

The surgeon then dissects around the area around the neck of the bladder. This is a very important part of the procedure because in this area are sited the muscles that control urination. If they are damaged, it is possible that incontinence will result.

Having dissected around the bladder neck, the surgeon will next remove the prostate itself. The bladder neck is then reconstructed. This is a very delicate and absolutely critical part of the procedure because if it is done incorrectly there may be subsequent scarring which can lead to the formation of a stricture or narrowing, thus causing many post-operative difficulties. A catheter is placed in the urethra and the urethra sewn around the catheter and on to the reconstructed bladder neck. This concludes the major part of the operation. The abdomen is then repaired and you are sent to the anaesthetic recovery room.

Surgey: after removal of the prostate.

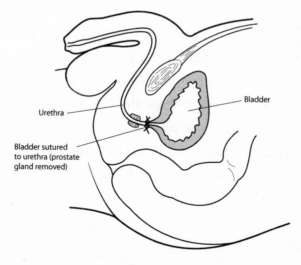

The period in the recovery room usually lasts two to three hours. When you have recovered from the anaesthetic you are sent back to the wards. On waking in the wards you will find a drip in your arm, a catheter in your penis and wound drains emerging from your abdomen. The latter are plastic tubes which drain the ooze of blood and serum from the prostatectomy bed.

Two or three days after the operation, the drains are shortened. It may be that the drains remain in place for a few more days if there is leakage from the abdomen. In uncomplicated circumstances the drains are taken out around the fifth post-operative day. The urinary catheter may remain in place for seven days or longer, commonly for two weeks. Antibiotics continue for between three and five days during the post-operative period. The Heparin is discontinued at the beginning of the second post-operative week, when you are up and about and may be at the point of being discharged home.

After the Operation

It takes a while to get back to normal. Don't expect to be at normal strength until at least three months after the operation. Take it easy, don't push yourself, and allow yourself to be looked after. Eat well, eat normally and don't go on a crazy diet because this affects wound healing. Enjoy alcohol in moderation, and gradually take on a regular pattern of exercise to get back to normal fitness. Do not exercise excessively, and always stop when your body tells you to, by means of muscular aches and pains. This is all common sense ... you know it's what you have to do.

Side-effects

Surgeons were initially very happy about the consequences of prostatectomy, but recently, prompted by oncologists and patient support groups, they have begun to look in more depth at the side-effects of surgery.

Impotence

It used to be thought that sexual function was preserved in the majority of patients after surgery, but this may have been because the surgeons did not ask their patients in detail about their sex lives and patients did not complain about the loss of their potency. In fact, potency may be dramatically affected by this procedure, and there is some evidence that up to 70% of men who are potent before radical prostatectomy are rendered impotent as a result of the operation, even though the procedure is nerve-sparing.

There is a degree of recovery of potency, which increases with months from surgery and there is hope that, as time goes by, sexual function will improve. Where specialist centres report their results, the most highly skilled surgeons will describe loss of potency in between 25% and 45% of men. This loss can be helped by Sidenafil, more commonly known as Viagra, which is a tablet that will benefit between 40% and 80% of patients with prostate cancer who have been rendered impotent by surgery. Remember, tell your doctor earlier rather than later that you're having trouble getting an erection – the later you leave it, the less likely Viagra is to work.

Other ways of dealing with loss of potency include the use

of a tiny pessary that can be based inside the tip of the urethra. This tiny application is called a *muse*, and it will also help between 40% and 80% of patients.

More radical alternatives include the use of prostheses. An inflatable device is surgically inserted within the penis and connected to a small reservoir in the groin. The penis can be made rigid by massaging the skin in the groin over the reservoir, which pumps fluid from the reservoir to the penis. Another alternative is to use a vacuum pump. A tube is placed over the penis. Air is pumped out and an erection achieved. It sounds easy and it's worth a go, but it's not particularly successful, and not really the candle-lit dinner approach. However, don't be put off trying this method.

Incontinence

The other complication of prostatectomy is incontinence, which affects the lives of up to 40% of men post-operatively. This problem tends to decrease with time and, at six months from surgery, 1% of patients will have complete incontinence while a further 20% will have minor problems. The problem usually consists of urinary dribbling when the man stands or coughs or laughs. In the unfortunate case where there is complete incontinence, the condition may require the patient either to wear an incontinence pad or to be catheterised.

Strictures

Problems caused by strictures are reported in between 5% and 10% of patients. These are due to scarring around the surgical join between the bladder and urethra, causing a slowness of urination. Rarely, a patient may be completely unable to urinate and have to go to hospital for catheterisation. If the problem is severe, further surgery may be needed. This is a minor procedure in which a very small cutting instrument is inserted into the urethra to cut away the stricture.

Results

The results of surgery for prostate cancer are somewhat biased because of the rigorous patient selection. We really do not have a clear knowledge of the benefits of surgery over other treatments because these have not yet been established by randomised clinical trials. The results of treatment are presented from single hospitals, but these have no current comparative basis.

Only the fittest and youngest patients are acceptable candidates for surgery. They have by definition very low PSA levels and should therefore have no spread of their cancer. However, this is not necessarily the case, as shown by microscopic examination of the operative specimens, which demonstrates that up to 50% of all patients selected for surgery do not have a curative procedure because the cancer had already spread before surgery. This is either due to the spread of cancer beyond the prostate across the excision margins because the surgeon has, unknowingly, cut through an area of cancer and left tumour behind at the time of operation, or because the tumour has spread to involve lymph nodes.

Leaving aside the importance that selection bias plays in skewing the results of surgery, the results that are obtained are generally good. Although the major factor that determines survival appears to be tumour grade, overall, between 65% and 85% of all patients appear to be cured by this approach.

The following are my views on patient selection for the radical surgery treatment option for patients with localised prostate cancer:

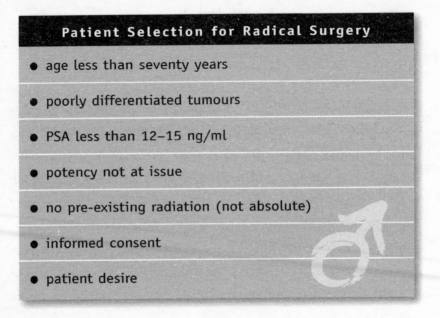

Patient Selection for Radical Surgery

- age less than seventy years

- poorly differentiated tumours

- PSA less than 12–15 ng/ml

- potency not at issue

- no pre-existing radiation (not absolute)

- informed consent

- patient desire

CHAPTER TEN

The Hormonal Treatment of Prostate Cancer

As explained in Chapter 1, the growth of the prostate gland is under hormonal control. In infancy the prostate is very small. It enlarges during puberty under the influence of testosterone, the male hormone, and a number of other hormones which include growth hormone and prolactin. The influence of these hormones combines so that in adult life the prostate is able to perform its normal function. In view of the influence of hormones on prostate growth it should come as no surprise that hormonal treatments are put into place to control prostatic cancer.

Hormone treatment is given to patients with large tumours in the prostate which are causing symptoms, or for the control of prostate cancer that has spread to the lymph nodes or bones. These treatments are designed to reduce the effects of testosterone, which is the most important of all of the factors stimulating prostate cancer growth.

The Basis for Prostate Cancer Treatment

The hormonal system is controlled by a cascade of molecular processes. These processes are very complicated, but it is important for you to understand them so that you know how hormone treatment for prostate cancer works.

The molecular processes begin in the brain. Here biological clocks, which are under the influence of time, light, mood and life cycle, respond to these influences by producing small chemical molecules called *neurotransmitters*. The neurotransmitters stimulate a glandular structure called the hypothalamus, which sits right in the centre of the brain and is positioned just behind the eyes. The hypothalamus, which can be described as the conductor of the endocrine orchestra, is the controlling organ for the body's hormones. Depending upon the frequency with which it receives the neurotransmitter signals from the cortex of the brain, and also upon the amount of neurotransmitter released, the hypothalamus responds in different ways, implementing the processes of puberty in both men and women and menstrual cycling in women.

Encased in a bony cave just below the hypothalamus is an endocrine gland called the pituitary, which is about the size of a large pea. Signals are sent from the hypothalamus down to the pituitary, either directly through nerve fibres or through blood vessels. The pituitary responds to these signals by producing hormones or by releasing other hormones sent from the hypothalamus and stored in its cells.

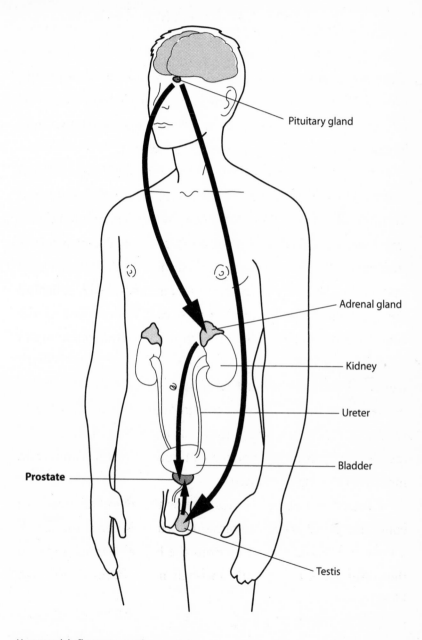

Pituitary gland

Adrenal gland

Kidney

Ureter

Bladder

Prostate

Testis

Hormonal influences on the prostate.

The most significant of the hormones produced by the pituitary for reproductive and sexual function are *luteinizing hormone* (LH) and *follicle-stimulating hormone* (FSH), which respectively control the manufacture of male hormones in the testes and stimulate the production of sperm. This manufacturing process is controlled by a hormone produced by the hypothalamus: *gonadotrophin-releasing hormone* (GnRH), which is also called *luteinizing hormone-releasing hormone* (LHRH). When luteinizing hormone and follicle-stimulating hormone are released from the pituitary they travel along the blood stream to the testes. Here they directly affect cell growth and metabolism, sparking the metabolic processes that lead to the production of testosterone, the male hormone, and sperm. The male hormone is made by specialised cells within the testes called *Leydig cells* and sperm is manufactured by cells called *germinal epithelium*. Testosterone is manufactured by a chemical process from cholesterol. Approximately 95% of all testosterone in the blood stream comes from the testes.

However, the same metabolic processes that lead to the production of testosterone in the testes also take place within the adrenal gland. This is a complex enzymatic chemical synthesis and involves many, many biochemical steps. These steps are controlled by hormonal feedback cycles which inhibit the release of the pituitary hormones. As part of this regulatory process, chemicals are released from the testes, travel back in the blood stream to the brain and decrease the release of luteinizing hormone and follicle-stimulating hormone from the pituitary. The control of hormone production is thus constantly reviewed by the biochemical control mechanisms that operate at a molecular level within cells, so that an imbalance of testosterone, luteinizing hormone and follicle-stimulating hormone should not occur.

The story does not end here, because testosterone is a relatively inactive hormone. To have its effects upon the tissues testosterone has to be altered biochemically within the cells where it works. The enzyme that causes this biochemical transformation is called *5-alpha reductase*. As a result of the action of 5-alpha reductase, testosterone becomes activated to *dihydrotestosterone* (DHT), the active male hormone.

Dihydrotestosterone binds to a protein called the *androgen receptor* within the cells where male hormones have their effect. The androgen receptor travels into the nucleus of these cells and then acts upon certain genes, stimulating them into producing chemicals that carry out the cellular processes. In other words, the effects of the male hormones take place through genes switched on by the male hormones. It is these genes that are responsible for some of the physical differences between men and women.

It is only by understanding these complicated hormonal actions that drugs to treat prostate cancer can be manufactured (*see diagram on page 98*). All hormonal treatments aim to negate the effects of testosterone on the tissues and they do so in a variety of different ways.

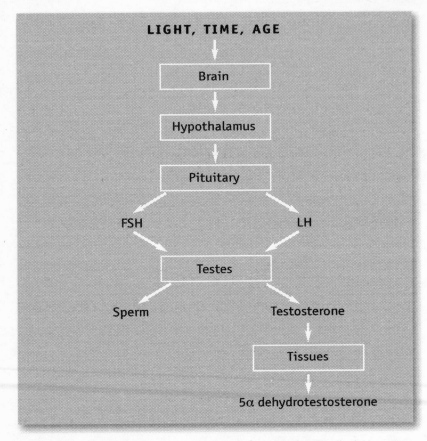

How male sex hormones and sperm production are controlled from brain to testes

How Hormone Treatments for Prostate Cancer Work

The history of prostate cancer treatment goes back many years. The reader should be encouraged rather than made miserable by the following historical descriptions, because over the last sixty years there have been so many improvements in treatment. These have produced hormone therapies that are patient-friendly.

The first attempts at treatment date from the end of the

nineteenth century, when an English surgeon castrated men with prostatic diseases and found that castration led to symptom relief. This work was largely forgotten until the early 1940s, when two Americans, Charles Huggins and Charles Hodges, popularised the first widely available treatments for prostate cancer. Huggins and Hodges went on to receive the Nobel prize for their work, which led to great medical excitement and even greater excitement on the part of patients who were relieved of their pain and urinary symptoms by the relatively simple treatments which will now be discussed.

Orchiectomy

Orchiectomy is the medical name for castration or the surgical removal of the testes. It is a relatively quick operation which can be carried out either under general anaesthetic or spinal anaesthetic. There are two types of orchiectomy: *total orchiectomy* and *subtotal orchiectomy*.

A total orchiectomy involves the removal of all testicular tissue, whereas a subtotal orchiectomy involves the removal of the hormonal and sperm-producing apparatus of the testes, leaving the capsule of the testes behind. This capsule becomes filled with blood. A scarring process then takes place during which the residual blood becomes fibrous. The scarring eventually gives the impression of a normal testicle within the scrotum. However, as the months and years go by the tissue left becomes absorbed and very little material remains.

Those in favour of orchiectomy as a treatment for prostate cancer argue that once the operation has been performed, it can be forgotten about because it is a procedure that is relatively quickly done and the patient does not have to take any medicines. This argument is all very well but it is difficult to forget that one's testicles have been removed. After a lifetime with them, most men become attached to their testes! As for the patient being able to forget about treatment of his cancer, modern work has shown that if a patient takes tablets in addition to having an orchiectomy his survival may be prolonged. So, in addition to the orchiectomy itself, there remains a twice-daily reminder of illness.

A second argument put forward by advocates of orchiectomy is that it is a cost-effective procedure. In other words, it is cheap. However, the operation is usually carried out while the patient is in hospital, and surveys have shown that the average period of hospitalisation for this procedure is ten days. As a hospital bed costs an average of £300 per day, the cost of orchiectomy is £3,000, which is comparable to the lifetime costs of any medical treatment for prostate cancer.

Orchiectomy is described as a relatively simple and straightforward procedure. To my mind it is neither simple nor straightforward. Moreover, there are effective medical alternatives that require no surgical procedure. Still, these matters remain within the area of patient choice and, having been properly informed about the options open to him, the patient may prefer this route.

Oestrogen therapy

Oestrogens have been used to treat prostate cancer for over sixty years. The main oestrogen given to patients for prostate cancer is *diethylstilboestrol* (DES), a synthetic female hormone. It works by blocking the release of luteinizing hormone-releasing hormone (LHRH) from the hypothalamus to the pituitary, which in turn stops the manufacture and release of luteinizing hormone (LH) from the pituitary to the Leydig cells in the testes, thus shutting off the production of testosterone. Treatment is generally given in the form of a tablet taken once or three times daily.

The results of treatment with oestrogens were not analysed in a statistically significant way until the mid-1960s, when the Veterans' Co-operative Group in the United States published the results of their findings on the treatment of patients with prostate cancer. The Veterans' Group consists of patients who were in the United States Armed Forces and are treated in the Veterans' Group of the United States hospitals that cares for ex-servicemen. The research group at the Veterans' Hospital showed that there was an increase in deaths from cardiovascular disease as a result of treatment of prostate cancer with oestrogen therapy.

The effects of oestrogens on the blood are very complicated. They include fluid retention and changes in the way that the blood clots, as a result of which blood pressure increases. Patients taking oestrogen are thus more liable to strokes and heart attacks. There is evidence that low dosages of oestrogen are just as effective as high dosages in the control of prostate cancer. However, the side-effects are similar even if small dosages are used, and this has been confirmed in many studies that continue to this day.

In addition to these serious cardiovascular consequences,

oestrogens have other effects. Approximately 30% of all patients treated with oestrogens develop quite significant gastrointestinal upset, consisting mainly of stomach pain, wind and nausea. There are mood changes too, and all patients suffer from swelling of the breasts, which may be very tender and most unpleasant. The breasts can also be quite profoundly enlarged. Since there are so many alternative treatments for prostate cancer, it seems unnecessary that patients are treated nowadays with female hormones.

This is also the view of doctors in many other European countries – a view which has led to the banning of oestrogen treatment on the grounds of its poor safety record in Germany. An argument for treatment with oestrogen in the United Kingdom is made on the basis of cost. Oestrogens are cheap, but I would argue the Gucci principle of cost: you get what you pay for, and cheap drugs are generally not as good as expensive ones. It is important to note that the effects of oestrogens on the heart remain, despite treatment with concomitant aspirin. I cannot recommend oestrogens as a treatment for prostate cancer, except under exceptional circumstances.

Anti-androgens

Anti-androgens are drugs that work by blocking the binding of testosterone and dihydrotestosterone to the androgen receptor. Amongst this class of drugs are Flutamide and Bicalutamide, otherwise known as Drogenil and Casodex, which are pure anti-androgens, and Cyproterone acetate, which is a complex anti-androgen. In contrast to oestrogens which block testosterone at the level of the hypothalamus, Flutamide and Bicalutamide do not lower testosterone. They block the effects of testosterone at a cellular level by stopping it from binding to the androgen receptor, a transport molecule that takes testosterone on a journey through the cell to its nucleus where it binds to DNA. Cyproterone acetate has this effect, and many other more complex roles in addition.

Flutamide was first introduced into the treatment of prostate cancer in the 1970s. Responses to treatment were said to be short-lived and it was noted that many patients suffered from very profound depression as a result of this drug's use. Flutamide is currently used in combination with other treatments for prostate cancer and only for very short periods on its own. Flutamide may have some other side-effects, which range in severity. The most common is diarrhoea, which occurs in 12% of all patients. It can be eased by reducing the dose of Flutamide but in many patients the diarrhoea is so intolerable that treatment has to be discontinued. In rare cases Flutamide may cause liver damage. This will manifest in changes in blood tests or, very rarely, in jaundice. If this develops then treatment must be discontinued. In a few very rare cases the side-effects of Flutamide on the liver can be such that death results.

Bicalutamide was introduced into the treatment of prostate cancer in the late 1980s. The introduction of this drug has been important for prostate cancer patients because it is a successful treatment without major side-effects. In fact, it has been argued that Bicalutamide can be used as a single treatment of prostate cancer. Bicalutamide is a purer anti-androgen than

Flutamide and has the advantage over many other treatments in that a proportion of patients will maintain potency despite therapy for prostate cancer. Approximately 40–50% of all patients treated with Bicalutamide as a single agent may have the good fortune to retain sexual potency. Many patients have nipple tenderness with Bicalutamide and this is sometimes treated with radiotherapy. Bicalutamide may also be used in combination with other treatments for prostate cancer.

Cyproterone acetate is a complicated drug in its biochemical effects upon the body. It may cause fluid retention and its use is associated with an increased risk of strokes and heart attacks. It may also have liver toxicity, and this side-effect occurs with a much greater frequency than the liver toxicity seen with other anti-androgens. For this reason it is advised that Cyproterone acetate is only used for a very short period of time. Clinical studies have shown that Cyproterone acetate is the best drug to prevent tumour flare – a term used to describe the initial and transient worsening of symptoms which is seen with treatment with LHRH agonists. The Committee of Medicines do not recommend long-term use of Cyproterone acetate.

Gonadotrophin-releasing hormone (GnRH) agonists

Doctors began using GnRH treatment in the early 1980s. My own interest in prostate cancer stems from this time when I was lucky enough to have been one of the first people to use these treatments to help patients with prostate cancer.

The GnRH agonists are synthetic molecules with similarities in structure to gonadotrophin-releasing hormone, the protein produced by the hypothalamus which stimulates the release and synthesis of luteinizing hormone and follicle-stimulating hormone from the pituitary. Repeated treatment with these agents desensitises the pituitary and causes a decrease in luteinizing hormone and follicle-stimulating hormone levels.

Treatment with these drugs was initially given by intranasal spray or continuous intravenous administration. (*Intravenous* means into a vein, as opposed to *subcutaneous*, under the skin.) Later, subcutaneous injections were given and in the mid-1980s these injections became available as once-monthly treatments. Subsequently three-monthly treatments have been developed. The drug remains under the skin of the injection site and gradually diffuses into the blood over a period of time, causing long-term suppression of the male hormones. The LHRH agonists are a humane and effective treatment of prostate cancer.

The more common side-effects associated with treatment include hot flushes, like those experienced by women around the time of menopause. Hot flushes can be mild or severe, infrequent or very frequent, but they can be treated. Their treatment includes other drugs, such as Clonidine and Medroxyprogesterone acetate, which themselves may cause some problems, or herbal remedies – which are rarely effective. The best treatment for hot flushes consists of keeping very cold, both during the day and at night in bed.

Other side-effects include anaemia and osteoporosis.

Testosterone is needed in males by the bone marrow to make blood, and so with low levels mild anaemia is common. Testosterone is required by bone to help it maintain its structure. Low testosterone weakens bone and this may be so significant that osteoporosis results. This is a condition that can lead to fractures, as often seen in elderly women. On average about 2% of bone protein is lost for each year of anti-androgen treatment. Evidence has emerged in 2001 that treatment with an infusion of a class of drug called a bisphosphonate given three monthly prevents this side-effect in prostate cancer patients.

LHRH agonists in combinations with anti-androgens

It was suggested in the early 1980s that, since the testis was not the only source of male hormones available to the body, it was important to eliminate all sources of male hormone. The other sources of these hormones are diet and the adrenal glands. From this was developed the theory of *total androgen blockage*, otherwise known as *maximal androgen blockade*.

The medical profession dealt with the concept with great scepticism. However, Fernand Labrie, the original protagonist of the theory, continued to promote his views so vigorously that, motivated by the furore created by his enthusiasm, the National Cancer Institute in the United States finally began a clinical trial comparing treatment with an LHRH agonist alone with LHRH agonist in combination with an anti-androgen. The results of this investigation were first published in 1989 and showed that there was a clear survival advantage to combination therapy.

The debate continues with regard to the use of combination treatment but a recent analysis, published in 2000, confirmed the advantage shown in the National Cancer Institute's study. This meta-analysis also showed that the advantage was small in terms of the patients' increased survival chance.

There are other advantages to combination therapy. These include the prevention of tumour flare and the opportunity for a further response to treatment should the cancer get out of control. This further response comes from stopping the anti-androgen.

Intermittent Hormonal Therapy

In an attempt to allow the return of potency, the practice of giving medical treatment intermittently was introduced in the late 1980s. It is possible that this may be as effective as continuous treatment in the control of prostate cancer, but further evidence for this is needed. Potency may take six months or so to return after discontinuing treatment, by which time PSA levels have started to rise and treatment needs to be restarted. This intermittent approach may, however, be psychologically disruptive for the patient.

Conclusion

In summary, hormonal therapy is given to patients with cancers that are either confined to the prostate or have spread.

Treatment has changed over the years and is now much more humane. Opinions are divided as to what is the Gold Standard, but it is my view that the combination of an LHRH agonist with an anti-androgen provides the best hope for prolonged survival.

CHAPTER ELEVEN

The Treatment of Recurrent Prostate Cancer

Unfortunately, for some patients prostate cancer may return after a period of control of the disease. This is described by doctors as *relapse* or *recurrence*. At relapse there are significant opportunities in a proportion of patients for a further response to treatment. Even though in some instances the long-term prognosis for the patient may not be all that great, in virtually all patients there are many opportunities for symptom relief.

It is absolutely essential for patients and their families to understand that patients with recurrence should not be considered to be 'terminal', and prolonged survival is very common. At this point in the patient's illness it is enormously important that there is an opportunity for a multidisciplinary approach to the disease. Indeed, the view is widely held that such a multidisciplinary approach should kick in right at the start of a patient's illness. It is my view that prostate cancer in relapse has to be managed by specialist cancer doctors, who will provide modern treatment such as chemotherapy and access to radiotherapy treatment machines.

The main problems for patients with recurrence are bone pain and urinary difficulties. Pain results from the spread of the cancer to bones, whilst urinary difficulties come because of re-growth to the prostate. Weight loss is unusual. It is also possible for patients with recurrence to become anaemic and require blood transfusion. Rarely, other complications may be seen. In some men, spread of the cancer to bones of the spine may lead to pressure on the blood supply to the spinal cord. This may critically imperil the spinal cord and cause a paralysis that may improve if treatment is instituted at an early enough point. The prostate may grow up and around the bladder, nipping off the ureters, which are the tubes that drain urine from the kidneys into the bladder. This may lead to kidney failure, which can be treated by putting little drainage tubes into the kidneys. I am sorry if this all seems frightening. Do remember that such problems are treatable, and by treatable we mean people can get better.

PSA in Relapse

Although on its own PSA may be a poor test for the initial diagnosis of prostate cancer, it is an excellent marker of prostate cancer response. It also reflects the activity of prostate cancer and gives advanced indication of progression of the tumour. PSA levels reach their low point shortly after the institution of treatment for prostate cancer. The lowest point will come two to three months after the beginning of hormonal treatment, six months after treatment with external beam radiotherapy, and up to five years after treatment with brachytherapy. The levels of PSA should become virtually unmeasurable within a few days of radical surgery.

At a median of thirteen months from the start of hormone treatment for prostate cancer, PSA levels begin to rise. Although this is a reflection of the increasing activity of prostate cancer, it is not a reflection of the symptoms that a patient will suffer from. In fact, symptoms will take an average of about a further two years to begin, and it is this wait for symptom development that understandably causes so much anxiety in patients with prostate cancer. It is important to note that this rise does not occur universally in all patients. This information relates to the average patient.

There is no evidence that early changes to treatment will have an effect on the overall survival of patients with prostate cancer and most doctors advise that changes in hormone treatment are reserved for symptom progression – that is, the treatment change is reserved for when it is needed. This situation is terribly difficult to live with and many patients will have so much anxiety around this issue that treatment change should be considered by clinicians when PSA levels rise.

Hormonal Therapies for Relapsed Prostate Cancer

A number of different treatments are available for patients with prostate cancer who experience a relapse. The simplest of all treatments and the most difficult to understand both emotionally and scientifically is the discontinuation of anti-androgen treatment with Flutamide or Bicalutamide. It seems extraordinary that patients should get better simply by stopping one of the drugs used to treat their condition, but this is the case and up to 40% of patients will improve by discontinuing treatment with Flutamide or Bicalutamide.

Unfortunately, this improvement is only temporary. The average period of time for which the improvement continues is about seven months, but many patients will get better again simply by restarting the Flutamide. The period of time for which the improvement continues is generally half that observed for the first response – i.e. three and a half months. It is important to note that the LHRH agonist should not be stopped, because there is some slight evidence that discontinuing the LHRH agonist will lead to a much more rapid progression of the cancer.

Steroids

The second hormonal treatment offered patients in relapse consists of steroids. Cortisone or Hydrocortisone in small doses will lead to a further benefit. This improvement occurs in between 10% and 20% of patients but, unfortunately, is for a limited period only.

Steroids in high dosages may be used for the complications of prostate cancer. Dexamethasone, which is a very powerful steroid, is given in high dosages for neurological complications. The most common of these is called *cord compression*, in which tumour presses upon the spinal cord and obstructs the blood supply to the cord. The nerves within the spinal cord then die and the patient becomes paralysed below the level of the obstruction. Treatment with steroids, if instituted early enough, will help this situation, but radiotherapy is also required. Radiotherapy effectively kills the tumour which allows the spinal cord to recover, whilst the steroids lead to a temporary shrinkage of the damaged area around the tumour cells.

Chemotherapy for Recurrent Prostate Cancer

As was explained earlier, the majority of patients with prostate cancer tend to be older men. Chemotherapy drugs may be toxic, and young patients are far more resistant to the toxicity and side-effects of chemotherapy than the elderly. For this reason, chemotherapy was not really given to patients with prostate cancer in the 1970s and 1980s. When it was, the side-effects were such that the treatment was often worse than the disease itself.

In the 1980s oncology practice started to change, with an emphasis upon the refinement of treatment so that the benefits remained whilst the side-effects were lessened. The most useful drug that became available at this time for prostate cancer patients was called Mitozantrone, which has the trade name of Novantrone. For patients whose quality of life is poor because of their symptoms, life quality can be improved by combining Mitozantrone with low dose steroids. Although this does not produce a major improvement in life expectancy, there are definite benefits to patients' well-being. The side-effects of treatment are minimal: nausea and vomiting are generally not seen, hair loss does not occur and patients very rarely have infections. The advantages of Mitozantrone and its lack of disadvantages have made this a very popular approach for recurrent disease.

Palliative Radiotherapy

Radiotherapy is one of the best treatments for the control of pain in prostate cancer. Many years ago treatment with radiotherapy was rather complicated and pain control was achieved by administering multiple treatments over a prolonged period of time. It was clearly unsatisfactory to treat pain over a period of two weeks, for it is always much better to spend time at home than in hospital.

Treatment with five sessions of radiotherapy was compared with more complex prolonged radiotherapy treatments and it was concluded that there was an equal effect on pain relief. Recently one single radiation treatment has been compared to three or five fractions and found to have exactly the same effect in terms of pain relief. So a treatment process that is virtually identical to having a single X-ray can be given to relieve pain. We do not feel, as doctors, that there is any rationale to more complicated radiotherapy treatment schedules.

The effects of radiation therapy on pain relief are gradual, generally peaking at two weeks. Where there are multiple sites of bone pain, involving either the lower body or upper body, *hemi-body radiotherapy* is given. That is, treatment is given to one half of the body, either the lower or upper half. Hemi-body radiotherapy may have more side-effects than a single treatment given to one small site, and may therefore cause more nausea. There is also risk of marrow suppression, which can lead to anaemia, bleeding or infection. Patients receiving hemi-body radiotherapy are pre-treated with modern anti-sickness drugs, and this controls nausea in up to 80% of all patients, and the other side-effects are really quite unusual.

Hemi-body radiotherapy can be repeated, but a period of time is required before re-treatment because the bone marrow will have been suppressed by the radiotherapy and needs time to recover. This recovery period is generally six weeks, during which time re-population occurs from bone marrow at other sites within the body.

Radioisotope Treatment

Radioisotope treatment has been available for many years but is increasing in popularity as a treatment for bone pain resulting from secondary spread of prostate cancer. One of the most commonly used radioisotopes is strontium. This is only given to patients with multiple sites of pain in the bones. It can be regarded as a slightly complicated way of giving external beam radiation.

The advantage of radioisotope treatment over hemi-body radiotherapy is that it goes to multiple sites within the body and is not confined to one half of the person. The perennial grumbles about the cost of treatment are raised in association with this means of therapy, but the cost equation needs to consider firstly the patient and secondly all of the other therapies that may be necessary should radioisotope treatment with strontium not be given. It should be noted that only a small minority of patients are suitable for such treatment.

Prostate Cancer and the End of Life

When prostate cancer has progressed and life expectancy is short, it is important for the patient and his family to know that there should be no pain and no suffering at the end. No medals are awarded for suffering and the patient with pain should take his painkillers in adequate amounts so that pain is controlled. Very strong medicines are available to control symptoms and fear, and doctors and nurses have been trained to prescribe and give these drugs with freedom. Relief of the patient's suffering is a profound priority.

The drugs that are given to control pain are constipating. There is current research in pharmaceutical companies directed towards finding non-constipating pain control treatments, but these are as yet at an early stage. Because strong pain killers are constipating it is essential to take laxatives and take them in sufficient amounts to prevent constipation. Macmillan nurses can help in all kinds of ways by advising on both how to increase strong painkillers and alleviate their side-effects with balancing doses of the right laxatives. These strong painkillers also cause nausea, but this usually is mild and lasts just a few days.

Many patients believe that they are not allowed to have alcohol whilst they are taking strong medicines, but this is not the case because many drugs mix very well with drink. Obviously one should be a little careful and find one's way at first. A little at a time to find what's right. Because you may find that the combination of opiates, such as MST, and large amounts of alcohol are either very jolly or terribly unpleasant, be careful but enjoy yourself.

Other Matters

This chapter has so far dealt with medical treatments for prostate cancer when it has returned, but there are many other significant issues that need to be addressed at this point in a patient's life. At this time, help and support are available from palliative care teams, Macmillan nurses, the Prostate Cancer Charity Helpline team, district nurses, and the patient's GP. It is the interaction of all of these people with the man who has recurrent cancer and his family that is so important.

This is an emotional time for the man with prostate cancer, who may be faced with a limited prospect. Many men do not wish to talk about their illness but rather want to carry on as they have always done. They find it unhelpful continually to dwell on the issues of pain and dying, and would rather just watch their grandchildren play from the quiet of an armchair or talk to old friends over a beer.

Everyone needs to find his own way at this time. For some patients it is important to have the peace of mind of knowing that their affairs are in order. They do not want those they leave behind to have the disheartening experience of sorting through piles of paper of uncertain importance. One of my dearest patients very sweetly left little notes for his wife throughout the house, and after he was gone she frequently turned up little words of advice that related to the areas of the house that she was exploring for light bulbs, fuses and electricity meters.

Rather strangely, this can also be a cathartic time. I have known many patients who have told their friends and relatives what they really think about them. In one case, one of my patients told members of his family that he had hated them all his adult life. Unfortunately for his relationships, he recovered from the doldrums and had to face these hated relatives at family weddings and Barmitzvahs!

Above all, this is a time for conversations with one's dearest loved ones. Although so much may be said without words, there still may remain a lack of clarity in the interaction, which I guess is my rather muddled way of saying that it's so good for husbands and wives, and fathers, sons and daughters to tell each other that they love one another.

CHAPTER TWELVE

Alternative Approaches
Complementary and Alternative Therapies, and Support Groups

When people are diagnosed with cancer they are frequently overwhelmed by a feeling of absolute powerlessness. For men this loss of power can be very difficult. They may, for the first time in their lives, be facing a situation where they no longer feel they are in control.

Many people with cancer wish to re-assert control over their lives. The field of alternative medicines and complementary therapies can be a wonderful support at this time, allowing patients to feel that they are doing something for themselves about their illness. The medicines are accessible, the complementary therapists approachable; all that patients require is money to purchase these props to take control again. For the majority, this is a great thing to do because it is psychologically enabling. It provides the patient with the comfort of regaining control, and having done this they can proceed through the trials of treatment.

Diet

Much has been made of the importance of diet in altering the outcome of cancer. Specialist centres have been set up to provide advice for patients – centres that strongly advocate dietary change. It is clear that there are enormous benefits from dietary approaches to malignancy, but in my view these approaches, although psychologically supportive, have no objective benefit in terms of limiting the spread of cancer. Diets that are without dairy produce and meat have their strong protagonists, but for most people it is awfully difficult to assume a vegan lifestyle. Vegan diets may cause weight loss and this can be very debilitating, both physically and psychologically, for the patient with cancer.

It is clear that a significant proportion of patients with cancer feel empowered by taking control of their diet, and the good spirit that this produces can help them through their illness. However, such dietary measures may be inappropriate for some patients once their cancer develops, because the quality of their lives can plummet. The man who is used to eating a good steak on a Saturday night enjoys life less by giving up his steak and chips.

But there are many definite gains from dietary approaches. These benefits often come as a result of the community that a patient finds as a result of going on a course at a centre that offers dietary advice. For the first time the patient with cancer will find himself surrounded by cancer patients who are seeking to improve upon the quality of their existence and fight the cancers they have. Such a community can give hope, a hope that comes from a sharing of the load, and hope from a shedding of the burden of being alone with cancer, of finding a way when lost.

Many patients I know who have gone to centres that offer dietary advice come away from their residential courses feeling that they have participated in a wonderful experience. They may alter their diet slightly or not at all as a result of this experience, but what they have benefited from is the experience of sharing their troubles with people – other cancer patients and the residential course staff – who have time to listen to them.

The Gerson Diet

Gerson was an American doctor who suggested that changing diet might control cancer. His diet, the Gerson diet, consists mainly of fruit and vegetables of organic origin. Dr Gerson recommended changes to the relative balance of the basic elements of diet; sodium intake is limited and potassium is encouraged. Coffee enemas are recommended and may be taken two or three times each day. The Gerson Clinic is alive and well, and patients are treated south of the border in Mexico. Some words of caution ... there is no evidence whatsoever that the Gerson diet is of value in the treatment of cancer, and many find the enemas very debilitating.

Vitamins

Our modern diets are hugely different from those of our biological ancestors, who ate uncooked food and far more vegetables and fruit than we do. Our ancestors' diets were also much richer in vitamins and trace elements. Our own bodies are unable to manufacture vitamins and trace elements and it is possible that our reduced consumption of these essential dietary components has contributed to the development of malignancy.

Many patients take vitamin and trace element supplements. Vitamin C and B complex are safe for you to take, as are recommended amounts of commonly occurring metals such as zinc, and trace metals, such as selenium. However, you should be extremely careful when taking Vitamins A, D and E, because in excess amounts these vitamins will cause very significant medical problems which can even be fatal. It is therefore very important to take the dosages recommended in the information leaflets that come with supplements.

Patients generally feel better for taking vitamins and there is no doubt that the improvement in morale that comes from taking vitamins is beneficial.

Teas

There has been much interest in the observation that cancer of the prostate is less common in people of Asian origin. Although the reason for this is thought to be purely dietary, there is a school of thought which has it that the use of herbal teas is part of the reason for the lower rate of prostate cancer in the Far East. Green teas, which are most pleasant, have become popular as a supplement for patients with cancer. The rationale for the protective influence of green tea may be that it has anti- oxidant qualities, reducing the availability of the 'free radicals' that possibly cause cancer. Free radicals are chemicals that carry a 'charge'. This charge can cause changes in the cells that come into contact with them, possibly the starting point for cancer development. Any foodstuff that has anti-oxidant qualities mops up these free radicals, reducing risk. It is said that the increased used of preservatives – anti-oxidants – in foods has led to the significant reduction in stomach cancer in the Western World.

Although it is very unlikely that green teas are protective or help make the cancer go away, there is no doubt that this is a reasonable and soothing approach to illness.

Complementary Therapies

Complementary therapies claim to treat the whole person – body, mind and spirit – and not just the symptoms of their illness. It is thought that this 'holistic' approach has benefits for the patient's general sense of well-being. Some complementary therapies, such as acupuncture and hypnosis, are reputed to be several thousand years old. Unlike conventional medical treatments which have a scientific basis, the majority of complementary therapies work in a mysterious way that eludes scientific investigation. Because of this lack of an evidence base, their efficacy in the treatment of illness is difficult to evaluate. This lack of proof is often put as an argument for a benefit!

Although many complementary therapies now have regulating bodies which ensure that therapists are properly trained and qualified, there are many unqualified and unregistered therapists who have set up in practice. If you are considering complementary treatment, it is recommended that you go to a qualified practitioner. If you have difficulty in finding one near you, contact the relevant regulating body for a list of qualified therapists in your locality. My own feeling with regard to acupuncture and hypnosis is entirely positive, and I will review these subjects in more detail later in this chapter.

Homeopathy

Homeopathic medicines have become increasingly popular in our modern society. According to homeopaths, an infinitesimally small amount of a compound restores balance and contributes to good health.

Homeopathy, which was developed by Samuel Hahnemann, a German doctor, some 200 years ago, claims to work on the principle of 'like cures like'. That is, if a substance creates the symptoms of a particular disease in a healthy person, then the same substance will cure that disease in a sick person.

Homeopathic remedies are prepared by the serial dilution of a substance thought to have some activity. One part of the original substance is diluted with 99 parts of a liquid solution, usually water. The mixture is then 'succussed' – i.e. rhythmically shaken – in a process which is claimed to 'potentise' the liquid solution. This starting solution, known as the 'mother solution', is successively diluted in the ratio of 99:1 until the desired potency for the remedy is reached. It is thought that these successive dilutions increase the medicinal activity of the original substance while reducing its toxicity. The final dilution is thought to confer healing properties. It is suggested that the diluted original chemical causes a change in the atomic structure of the water in which it is diluted. We are not able to measure this effect on water.

Because the final remedy contains no measurable trace of the original substance, it is very difficult to establish a scientific rationale for the curative effect of homeopathic remedies. How is it that a grain of salt diluted 14 billion times could be a potential cure for cancer? Despite this reservation, there is no doubt that homeopathy has been beneficial for many patients. This may in part be due to the psychological support offered to patients by a visit to a homeopath, a support whose benefit cannot be trivialised or minimised.

Acupuncture

Acupuncture is an ancient form of Chinese medicine. According to acupuncturists, the health of an individual depends on the harmonious flow of energy along a grid-like system of invisible lines, called *meridians*, within the body. When an imbalance or blockage of energy occurs, disease results. The acupuncturist aims to restore the body's natural energy balance by inserting very fine needles at specific points, known as *acupuncture points*, along the appropriate meridian. Acupuncture has been used successfully to control pain and nausea.

There are no specific qualifications required to set up practice as an acupuncturist. However, the British Medical Acupuncture Society offers training courses and a Certificate of Accreditation, and provides helpful regulation of the practice. It is clearly the case that people can feel great after a trip to the acupuncturist. It is also clear that acupuncture leads to measurable chemical changes – fluctuations in the body's endorphins (naturally occurring opium-like chemicals) – and that these changes may be the biochemical basis for the effects of acupuncture.

Reflexology

In this technique pressure is applied to specific zones on the soles and tops of the feet. Each zone corresponds to a zone in the body, and it is suggested that energy flows along connections between the two zones. However, it is unclear what these 'connections' are. Massage in particular areas of the foot has been used to help patients with cancer. Many people feel calmed by the treatment, which is gentle and soothing. It is thoroughly recommended for cancer patients. In our own cancer unit we employ reflexologists and they have been of great benefit, as evinced by the queues for their services!

Aromatherapy

Aromatherapy involves the use of aromatic oils, which are gently massaged or rubbed into the skin of patients with cancer. The action of having the oils massaged into your skin is an enormously relaxing and wonderful process. The oils themselves are soothing and the benefits to the patient from this process quite clear. We are convinced of the benefit of aromatherapy and also employ an aromatherapist within our own hospital department, and have done so for many years. A succession of aromatherapists have helped many of our patients with cancer and made their load much easier to bear.

Currently, aromatherapists and other massage therapists are not subject to any formal regulation. Attempts have been made to regulate this practice, mainly through massage therapy schools. The effects of aromatherapy on patients with cancer have been investigated. The relaxation and calmness that come from this technique have been found to reduce anxiety and improve life quality.

Hypnosis

The history of hypnosis is ancient, dating back in many forms over many millennia. The techniques of hypnosis were introduced into medicine by Charcot, an eminent French physician, and then brought into the popular conscience by Mesmer, to who we owe the verb 'to mesmerise'.

Hypnosis has become a very useful medical tool in modern times for the treatment of mental disorders, such as phobias and anxiety. In cancer, too, it has a significant role and can be a wonderful tool to help people through their illness, providing the patient with useful techniques for relaxation and visualisation for dealing with pain or for coping with the nausea and vomiting that may come from cancer chemotherapy.

Patients are taught to enter a state of relaxation by the use of methods that generally involve a combination of eye fixation and progressive muscular relaxation. This is a highly recommended way of dealing with pain and nausea. The amount of pain a patient experiences can also be helpfully reduced: the patient's perception of pain is increased by his or her anxiety, and it can be decreased by hypnosis. Patients can also be taught to imagine in a hypnotic state that their tumours are being nibbled away by fish floating in their blood streams. This visualisation encourages the patient to feel that he's getting better with treatment and that his own mind is controlling the tumour's growth. This is empowerment. This helps the patient to take back control from a cancer that has disempowered him.

Distant Healing

There are healers within our community, and people who have psychic power (whatever that means and whatever that is) do have a role to play in cancer care. For a long time we had, working in association with the Cancer Centre at our hospital, a man who believed that he was a psychic healer. He would think about the patients who were treated in our Centre and think positively that they were getting better. Well, we were grateful for his assistance.

Psychic Surgery

The practitioners of psychic surgery delve into abdomens and produce what appear to be tumorous growths, miraculously removing these growths without leaving any evidence that the abdomen has been opened. There is no cut, there are no scars and the psychic surgeon has cured the patient of his cancer!

Psychic surgeons, who practise their occult discipline in the Far East, particularly in Indonesia and the Philippines, achieved some notoriety in the 1980s. Patients in search of a cure would travel from around the world to see these charlatans. But although this charade has led to no cures, it *has* benefited some people: the psychic surgeons who have managed to extract significant amounts of money from the wallets of poor people desperate for life. The tumours miraculously removed by the psychic surgeons have been found to be pieces of chicken and the entrails of pigs. A horrid deception.

Alternative Medicines

The testing of alternative and herbal medicines is much less rigorous than the testing of conventional medical products. The reason for this is that complementary medicines are classified as food products and so the tests applied are those used to investigate foodstuffs. These tests require only a minimal level of safety investigation and do not take into account any scientific evaluation of medical efficacy. In other words, no scientific proof has to be obtained that these complementary drugs actually work, and this is in direct contrast to the rigorous testing that is carried out on conventional drugs made by the pharmaceutical industry.

Researchers have found in alternative medicines both toxic compounds that may cause side-effects and also the natural equivalents of drugs that are used to treat prostate cancer. Some of these substances include steroids and female hormones and will by themselves lead to an improvement in PSA levels or sometimes in symptoms.

The reader should understand that the pharmaceutical industry and conventional medicine are not at loggerheads with alternative medicine. Indeed, you may be surprised to learn that the pharmaceutical industry turns to the natural world to source the drugs that we use to treat illness: chemotherapy agents are derived from pine needles harvested from the Pacific Yew, from algae taken from the deep sea of Japan, and from the periwinkle plant. We have taken from the natural world what works ... and put it to work.

Putting any argument to one side, the following are some of the more common alternative medicines used for patients with cancer.

PC Spes

One of the most popular of recent alternative medicines has been PC Spes, a product which has significant activity in patients with prostate cancer. This is because it contains plant equivalents of diethylstilboestrol, a synthetic female hormone used to treat prostate cancer. PC Spes is made up of eight plant extracts, including chrysanthemum, liquorice and ginseng.

Medical studies have shown that patients do improve with PC Spes. However, this improvement comes with a downside. There is toxicity, patients develop breast swelling and they have indigestion. These are symptoms that are common in patients taking diethylstilboestrol (DES) and they are one of the reasons why treatment with diethylstilboestrol is only rarely prescribed nowadays.

Shark fin

Shark fin extract is sold to patients with prostate cancer, and indeed to many patients with other malignancies. The theoretical basis for the use of shark fin is that sharks, to our knowledge, do not develop cancer. Shark fin extract is used to treat patients with cancer in the hope that, like sharks, they will not have any tumours.

Tumours require the nutrients that are contained in blood in order to develop and grow. They also produce chemicals that lead to the development of blood vessels from the surrounding normal tissues. This new blood supply allows cancers to expand. It is thought that sharks' cartilage possibly contains a factor that inhibits the development of these new blood vessels, thus inhibiting the supply of the tumour with nutrients.

Shark cartilage is very expensive and produces major benefits to the companies that manufacture the shark fin extracts. There is absolutely no scientific evidence that it is of benefit to cancer patients and, quite frankly, the real sharks are not in the water or the medicine bottle. They are on dry land, cynically taking advantage of the sick.

Almond kernels

Extracts of almond kernels have achieved some notoriety as a potential treatment for cancers. These alternative medicines were investigated by the National Cancer Institute in the United States. No benefit was shown for cancer patients. However, almond kernel extracts do have some theoretical basis for their activity: they contain cyanide, which is a cellular poison.

Bromelin

Bromelin, an enzyme that breaks down proteins, is isolated from the fruit of *pseudananas macrodontes*, a species of plant closely related to the pineapple. Bromelin has been used to treat patients with ulcerative colitis. Experimental work has shown that this compound produces an improvement in cellular immune competence – in other words, it is a boost to the immune system. To date there is no scientific evidence of its activity in cancer, but it certainly is an interesting compound.

Iscador

The use of Iscador as a treatment for cancer was pioneered by Rudolph Steiner, the founder of Theosophy. An extract of mistletoe, Iscador is a poison and has measurable effects upon the bone marrow. Patients who take it may develop anaemia or low levels of white blood cells or platelets, and subsequently may require blood transfusion or be at risk from infection or bleeding. There is absolutely no scientific evidence of its efficacy in the treatment of cancer and considerable evidence that Iscador has deleterious effects.

Saw Palmetto

Extracts of the herb saw palmetto (*serenoa repens*) are widely used. Proper analyses have shown that this works to improve urinary symptoms. It is one of the components of PC Spes. It reduces symptoms by about 25%.

Essiac

Essiac is a blend of a number of different herbs, including Indian rhubarb, sorrel, slippery elm and burdock. It is suggested that essiac stimulates the immune system and improves life quality. However, there is no significant evidence of its effects in cancer.

Support Groups

Support comes in many shapes and in very many forms, from the hospital porters and cleaning staff, nurses and doctors, neighbours, friends, family and colleagues. Support comes from talking and listening, from a kiss, from a cuddle. Formalised support networks, ranging from telephone helplines to patient groups or residential courses, are also widely available. I describe some of these organisations below. Further information and details of how to contact them are provided in Additional Information at the back of this book.

CancerBACUP

This organisation was started by Vicky Clement Jones, a wonderfully clever and determined doctor, who developed ovarian cancer. Vicky felt that patients were unable to obtain adequate information about their cancers and set up CancerBACUP with Maurice Slevin, a doctor who specialised in the treatment of ovarian cancer. This has become a major provider of information for patients and, through Maurice's continued marvellous efforts, patients can obtain telephone advice on cancer treatment. CancerBACUP is now hoping to develop hospital-based, walk-in information centres.

Bristol Cancer Centre

The Bristol Cancer Centre was set up by a group of patients

and doctors, some of whom had cancer. The Centre pioneered different approaches to cancer, championing alternative, homeopathic and dietary methods. Patients come from around the country to take part in weekend or weekly residential courses, where they are encouraged to share experiences with other patients in groups led by counsellors. The Bristol diet has been much publicised. It is a vegan diet that aims to put back a balance in the lives of cancer patients.

Macmillan

The Macmillan Service has gone from strength to strength over the last decade. Macmillan nurses are well known for their importance in symptom relief for cancer patients, but the Macmillan Service also provides a patient helpline and funds cancer doctors who are both hospital and community based.

The Prostate Cancer Charity

The Prostate Cancer Charity was set up in the mid-1990s to provide support for patients, to lobby for change in both the media's and government's perception of prostate cancer, and to fund basic research. The Charity has met with some success: a patient information service has been set up, trained nurses are available on a helpline, information booklets have been written and central government has increased prostate cancer research funding from £78,000 in the year 1996/7 to a projected £4.2 million in the year 2003/4. The Charity has started to fund prostate cancer specialist nurses to work in hospitals to support patients through their illness.

Summary

Everyone finds their own way to cope. Every day is a special day and a triumph to get through. Every moment can be made better by the way you feel, and the way that you feel depends upon not only the treatment you receive but also the support that you have around your treatment. These supports, whether they are homeopathic, provided by hypnosis, or by vitamins and diet, are all appropriate.

CHAPTER THIRTEEN

The Patients' Stories

In earlier chapters I described the various treatment options available to the patient with prostate cancer. Different options suit different people, and the final choice depends upon the personality of the patient and his interaction with his family and doctors. The following stories illustrate how a variety of patients went about making their choice, the questions they asked and the factors that led to them deciding on which option was best for them.

1. Brachytherapy

Gerald was 52 years old when he came to see me. He was a successful accountant in a multinational company, where he was one of 14,000 global partners. Health checks were provided as part of the care package offered by the company to its employees. These checks, which were carried out annually in employees over fifty years of age, consisted of an interview by a doctor, a physical examination and some blood tests. Amongst the blood analyses performed in these checks was the PSA test.

Gerald was advised by letter that his PSA result was raised, at 7.6 ng/ml. He showed the letter to his wife, Madeleine, who had been a hospital dietician before giving up work to raise her family. The children had grown up and she had returned to work in a health club as an aromatherapist and dietary specialist. She was into health foods and alternative medicine, counselling the members of the club on dietary deficiencies and giving all-round good advice.

When they made an appointment to see their doctor, he explained to Gerald and Madeleine that, at that sort of level, there was a 25% chance that Gerald might have prostate cancer, but also 75% chance that there would be nothing wrong, except perhaps for benign enlargement of the prostate or a touch of prostatitis.

After discussion of the situation with the doctor, an appointment was made for Gerald to see a urologist at the local hospital. The urologist told him and Madeleine that he saw a lot of people like Gerald and that raised PSA results seemed to cause much more trouble than they were worth because only a small percentage of patients had tumours. He added that the clinic was almost overwhelmed with what he called 'PSA-itis'. In the circumstances, there were two options for Gerald to consider. The first was the 'do nothing' option. The second was to arrange for a biopsy to be done. This second option would at least let them know what they were dealing with.

When he had finished explaining what the options involved, the urologist asked them what they wanted to do. Madeleine knew immediately what to do. She said that they would like to go home and have a chat about things. She thanked the doctor, and as she and Gerald were preparing to leave the consulting room she asked if there was anywhere she could go for more information. He replied that he wasn't too sure. The couple left the clinic, making an appointment to be seen again a week later.

At home they discussed the problem and Madeleine immediately set about changing her husband's diet. Gerald started to eat an awful lot of pizzas and carrots, consumed buckets full of vitamins and cart loads of selenium tablets. By the end of the week the couple had decided that it was better to know what they were dealing with, because then at least they could confront the issues with some knowledge of the condition. Somehow the known was less scary than the unknown.

The urologist arranged for Gerald to have a transrectal ultrasound and biopsy, which was carried out seven days after his clinic appointment. It was very undignified, Gerald thought, as he wiggled into position so that the ultrasound probe could be inserted into his rectum. Just before taking the biopsy, the radiologist told Gerald to brace himself because it could sometimes be uncomfortable. Gerald felt a dreadful jolt as the needle entered his prostate. The procedure was repeated six times and some of the insertions were very painful whilst others were not felt at all. Gerald got up from the examination couch and got dressed. He needed to go to the lavatory and when he wiped himself he was surprised to find blood on the lavatory paper.

At home that evening Gerald began to feel very unwell. It was as if he had the most frightful bout of flu. He phoned his GP, who came out to see him. His doctor suspected that Gerald had got an infection from the biopsy and they needed to get him back into hospital. Gerald was hospitalised for five days, during which time he was treated with intravenous antibiotics.

When Gerald and Madeleine next saw the urologist, he apologised, explaining that it was very unusual to get this sort of infection. He was right. Less than 1% of patients who have transrectal ultrasound guided biopsies have infections as a result of the procedure.

The urologist apologised again when he told them that there was a little bit of cancer in Gerald's prostate. When the couple asked him exactly what he meant, the doctor replied that there was a little bit of tumour in one of six cores of tissue taken from the prostate gland.

Madeleine said that they had been looking at the information booklets and had gathered that a lot depended upon the appearance of the tumour under the microscope. The doctor commented that she seemed to be remarkably well informed. The tumour was of moderate grade.

When Madeleine asked him about the Gleason grade, the doctor informed them that it was 2 + 3. He explained to Gerald that this meant the tumour had a relatively good outlook and things should be fine. He then told them that there were three options. The tumour could be watched, or Gerald could have surgery, or he could be treated with radiation therapy, of which there were two types.

The couple had read the Prostate Cancer Charity's information booklet about prostate cancer and understood what the options were. But they also understood that there was no clear idea as to what they should do in this situation. Even the doctors themselves were not quite sure exactly what the right way was to treat this condition.

The doctor agreed with them and said that he would tell

them about the surgery, but would send them to see a colleague of his, an oncologist, who could give them an idea about the other options. In the end, though, the choice was up to Gerald because doctors were uncertain as to the best way to manage the condition.

So Gerald went off to discuss the options of observation and radiotherapy with the oncologist, but still couldn't make up his mind what to do. He felt relatively calm about the situation and didn't spend too much time thinking about it. His wife, however, was very active in the way that she dealt with his tumour and intensified her efforts at homeopathic and alternative medical approaches. Meanwhile Gerald longed for a steak!

Eventually Gerald and Madeleine decided that they would opt for brachytherapy. They felt that the treatment would stand the best chance of curing Gerald's condition with the least side-effects. Gerald went through treatment this year with little in the way of side-effects and currently is well.

2. Watchful Waiting

Ron was 75. He owned a building business which had plenty of employees and specialised in modernising homes. Ron still worked and was actively involved in the day-to-day management of the business. He visited clients and talked about their needs, whether it be a new kitchen, a garage or general decoration. He would price up the job and then set his team the work. He was on site most days, supervising plumbers, electricians, plasterers, carpenters and painters and decorators. His wife, Susan, who was 65, was in the business with him. She did the books and made sure the men were paid.

Ron went for a regular annual medical run by a private health insurance agency, which Susan had insisted that he have if he wanted to carry on working. The blood tests carried out at the medical included a PSA test. After one medical Ron received a letter from the screening service suggesting that one of the blood test results was abnormal and that he needed to contact his family doctor about this. Ron was terrified and was all for ignoring the letter. Susan insisted that he did something about it. As Ron refused, she rang up and made the appointment for the doctor to see him.

Dr Green had been their doctor for forty years. He had seen them through the early stages of their marriage, their children, little crises, big crises, and the family regarded him as their friend. Every Christmas Ron took pleasure in dropping round to the surgery and leaving a bottle of malt whisky for his family doctor. When Ron and Sue went to their GP's surgery, Dr Green explained that the PSA test result was a little high. In his view there was very little to worry about, but just to be sure Ron ought to go and see a urologist. An appointment was made at the local hospital. Ron wanted to go through the NHS – he believed in it.

Six weeks later, Ron and Sue had their appointment in urology outpatients. The surgeon performed a rectal examination of Ron's prostate and then explained that, in his view, there was very little to worry about. The PSA result had come back at 10 ng/ml and this was a little bit over the normal value for Ron's age, but this was unlikely to be a problem. Besides, Ron had no symptoms from his prostate.

As Ron and Sue collectively breathed a rather large sigh of relief, the urologist went on to say that Ron's prostate had felt a little lumpy when he had examined him. He suggested that Ron should go for a biopsy and explained what this would involve.

Some two weeks later, Ron and Sue arrived at the X-ray department of their local hospital and ultrasound guided biopsies were performed. Ron found the experience uncomfortable but not too awful, embarrassing but not too miserable. Ron collected his thoughts and his trousers together and felt an immediate need to go to the loo. In the loo he was a little concerned to note that he was passing blood, but this wasn't painful. He had been warned by the radiologist that this might occur.

Another two weeks went by and then Ron and Sue went back to hospital for a review of the biopsy results. The urologist leaned forward in his chair and told them he was sure that everything was going to be fine, but he had to let them know that there was a minor abnormality in the biopsy, a tiny little focus of cancer.

Sue asked the doctor what he meant by 'a focus'. The urologist explained that it was just a little spot and nothing to worry about. Many people had these spots in their prostate and the evidence seemed to be that not much harm came from them.

Sue and Ron couldn't quite understand how it could be that having a cancer was something that really wouldn't cause a problem. In their minds having cancer was linked with certain death, and death within a very short period. The urologist did his best to reassure them. He explained that not all cancers are bad cancers, and that Ron's was a very mild form of cancer. If it were left alone over the next ten to fifteen years, there was only a 10% likelihood that it would cause Ron any trouble at all. If it did cause trouble, it could be deal with when it occurred.

Ron and Sue left the clinic and did a lot of thinking and talking. They discussed the situation on their way home, and at home, at work, with their friends, and with the various support agencies They went back to their GP and talked over the situation with him. He recommended that they see an oncologist for a second opinion. They did so and were very reassured by his explanation of their situation. They understood what the surgeon was talking about. He explained that the cancer was a mild one and would not affect their lives. Ron didn't need any treatment because it was not necessary.

Ron had no symptoms. He didn't want to have radiotherapy or surgery. He was happy doing without any active treatment. But there was one caveat, he needed to be followed up by the doctors just so that they could all see that the cancer did not worsen. Ron knew that if his situation changed he might need therapy and that regular monitoring was important.

Ron and Sue lived happily together over the next few years. At first they went for three-monthly check-ups to an oncology outpatient clinic, but gradually this period was extended until they went on a six-monthly basis. When he was 78, Ron gave up work and led a happy retirement. He died when he was 85. He died suddenly in his sleep, in the middle of the night, of what was thought to be a stroke. Over the whole period of his continued follow-up, he had had no symptoms from his prostate cancer and had not had to go through any active treatment.

3. External Beam Radiotherapy

Another of my patients was a business man called Harry. He had gone through the same routine screening tests as Ron and Gerald. Harry was 62 and leading an active and busy life when moderately differentiated Gleason 3 + 4 tumour was found in three of six of his biopsy cores. Harry's response was quite different from Ron's. He decided immediately that he wanted treatment; he didn't want to have anything complicated or fussy, just the standard treatment for his condition. He knew a little about surgery. One of his best friends had had a radical prostatectomy, and had regretted it because he had been bothered by quite severe side-effects from the operation. Harry's friend had become incontinent and impotent.

Harry had radiotherapy over six weeks and developed a little cystitis at the end of it. When he urinated it felt as though he was passing broken glass rather than urine, but the symptoms soon resolved. He also had some diarrhoea for a fortnight, going to the loo about ten or twelve times a day. His anus became sore and he ended up having to wash his bottom rather than wipe it, and he applied almond oil to his tail end to ease the soreness. But the diarrhoea started to improve when treatment stopped. During the whole period of treatment he worked, coming first thing in the morning for his radiotherapy treatment and then going off to his office in the city.

Unfortunately, two years after the completion of radiation

treatment there was a relapse. Harry was found to have raised PSA levels. He had some back pain and proceeded to have a bone scan. This showed spread of his cancer and he is now on hormonal therapy, but quite well. He is being treated with single agent bicalutamide (Casodex). He has unfortunately become impotent but is coping with this by using Cavajet. Viagra and Muse didn't work for him.

4. Surgery

Jack was a 68-year-old solicitor. His partner Jan was 47. Over a period of one year Jack had developed some minor urinary problems, getting up at night to pass water more often than he should. He went to his GP, who examined him and measured his PSA level. This came back as elevated beyond the normal range for his age. The normal range of results for PSA changes with age. A normal level of up to 3.5 ng/ml might be expected for a sixty-year-old but this increases to 6.5 ng/ml for a man of seventy years. Jack decided against any intervention at a very early stage and refused even to have a biopsy. It seemed that the couple's sex life was very important to them and Jack wanted nothing to compromise this. Eventually his urinary symptoms became a little more severe, so he had a biopsy which showed him to have a poorly differentiated Gleason 4 + 4 tumour. He had a surgical opinion and was convinced that the operation would be a good idea. Surgery was undertaken and within a week he was out of hospital. The catheter was removed at two weeks and he recovered well.

The surgeon who had carried out the procedure was a very

talented and modest man who had spent many years perfecting the technique and had reported his personal results in a series of over 300 patients. Two or three months after the operation Jack was entirely continent and cured of his urinary symptoms. Four months after the operation his sex life had returned to normal. Jack was a happy man.

5. Hormone Therapy

Colin had never married. He had always wanted to, but somehow never found the right person. He worked hard all his life and ended up as a quality supervisor in a plastics manufacturing business. Just as he was coming up to retirement he started to notice that things were not quite right. He had begun to get up at night, waking three or four times and rushing to the loo to pass just small amounts of urine. During the day he was embarrassed at work by having to leave the production line and go the lavatory, at first every hour, then every quarter of an hour. Something was definitely wrong. And one day at work he was unable to pass water at all. He went to the loo a few times but nothing happened. His stomach became tight and uncomfortable, and finally so uncomfortable that he went to the casualty department of his local hospital.

There he was examined and found to be in what is called 'retention' – that is, his flow of urine was completely obstructed. The examining doctor put some anaesthetic jelly into his urethra, inserted a catheter, and the agonising bursting sensation was immediately relieved. Colin was admitted to hospital from casualty and, after a couple of days, had biopsies of his prostate, which unfortunately showed him to have prostate cancer. His PSA level was very high at 800 ng/ml. Biopsies of the prostate showed him to have a poorly differentiated Gleason 5 + 5 tumour. Colin went on to have a bone scan which showed spread of his cancer to involve bones. A CT scan was performed and this showed enlargement of glands within his stomach.

Colin was quite naturally distraught. He was comforted by family and friends and had the good fortune to be living with his sister, who spent hours sitting and listening to him talk about his illness and his concerns that he would never, ever get better. She reassured him that he would, and her simple, straightforward support helped him through the early days of his illness.

Colin was started on some Flutamide tablets which, as the doctor explained, were given as part of a treatment pro-gramme for his prostate cancer. After a week of taking tablets, he was given an injection. The doctor told him that this would last three months and that he would need to be on the three-monthly injection treatment for the rest of his life. Colin asked about the tablets and whether or not he would need them too. He also asked how long the catheter would be needed. The doctor explained that, on balance, it was thought that the tablets did help, and that the combination of tablets and injec-tions provided the best hope for survival. After a period of three months, the treatment would have shrunk the prostate to a sufficient extent that there would be a good chance that Colin would be able to urinate again without the need for a catheter.

Colin went home and pretty soon began to feel much better. He had noticed over the previous month that he had developed what seemed to be arthritis, but with the treatment it appeared that the symptoms of arthritis were going. After a period of six weeks they had gone completely. Colin mentioned this to the doctors in clinic, who explained that the 'arthritis' symptoms were in fact symptoms from the spread of the cancer to his bones. Colin was asked in clinic whether he would like to talk about the outlook for his condition. But, after some discussion, he said that he didn't really want to know because he felt the knowledge would affect him in that he would be counting down his days. Besides, he knew that he could only be given an average and that, in real terms, there is no such thing as an average.

After three months of hormone treatment Colin was admitted to the day ward at the hospital and the catheter was removed. He was very pleased to be able to urinate normally again, released from the catheter and the leg bag that had so dominated his recent life. Colin is currently completely well, some two years after the initial diagnosis. He has taken early retirement and is happy enjoying so many of the things that he had been unable to do during his working life.

6. Alternative Medicine

Andy was 52 years old and owned a property company. He specialised in buying old properties, renovating them and re-selling them. His company had done very well in the late 1990s and he was comfortably off.

Andy was from the north of England; he was competitive in his work and blunt in his dealings with people. All his life he had known what he wanted, and he had got it. That is, until he developed metastatic prostate cancer. This was something that Andy most definitely did *not* want. He felt that he had lost control of his life to prostate cancer. Doctors were telling him what to do and what was best for him, and in his adult life nobody had ever done this before.

Andy was treated with once-monthly injections of leuprorelein (Prostap) by his GP and he took flutamide (Drogenil) tablets three times a day. There were some side-effects from the medicines. Initially the tablets had given him some diarrhoea, so he had reduced the dose and when the diarrhoea had gone away he was able to increase his dose again without harmful side-effects. Andy also suffered badly from hot flushes. These occurred three or four times during the day, stopping him in his tracks. He became red and sweaty, shivered, and then the attacks passed. In the night the hot flushes awoke him every hour and gave him a really hard time.

He was prescribed Clonidine by his GP to help with the flushes, but the tablets didn't work and put his blood pressure up. He was given Atenolol and this failed to help. He was then given a small dose of Medroxyprogesterone acetate, which Andy knew was a female hormone used by doctors to treat menopausal flushing. This miraculously cured his flushes.

Andy was angry about his fate. He had been looking forward to a happy and long life, a life in which he enjoyed himself and enjoyed the rewards of his life of labour. He was used to taking matters into his own hands and he certainly wasn't going to take things as they were. He was definitely not going to let the cancer win. He was going to help himself, and he did.

Andy read extensively about prostate cancer and the help that could be obtained from vitamin and mineral supplements. He investigated homeopathy and all alternative medicines. He bought shark cartilage capsules and vitamin E supplements, selenium and zinc tablets, and changed his diet so that he became a vegan and took a lot of saw palmetto. He eschewed dairy produce, ate no meat or milk and took an enormous amount of pleasure in cooking for himself. His wife was amazed by his culinary triumphs, and she changed her diet too.

The intensity which Andy had previously applied to his work was now redirected towards finding a cure for himself and trying to sort things out so that he could beat the illness. He modified his work style. He devolved the responsibilities of his job to three other senior employees within the company. He no longer went to work for twelve hours each day but, rather, popped in three times a week.

A turning point in his life came from a visit to the Bristol Cancer Centre. He booked himself in for a residential weekend and there, in the company of other patients – people with breast cancer, ovary cancer, prostate cancer, and lung cancer – he found a community. In the doctors and support therapists he found a group that cared and professionals that had time for him. Andy found that he was no longer alone. He realised with great relief that there were other people like him and, knowing this, took strength from the fact that there were others who were equally determined to change their lives and conquer their illness.

Finding a new family was the turning point for Andy. It was such comfort to him to know that he was not alone.

At Bristol, Andy was taught to meditate. He was taught hypnosis and the techniques of visualisation, and with these skills he felt calmness and tranquillity. And so it was that out of his experiences with cancer Andy really changed. He found a new strength and focus and was able to face the knowledge that he had cancer and deal with it.

Andy is currently well. It takes him about 20 minutes each morning to take all his tablets. He has stopped the coffee enemas because he felt that they were ridiculous. But he still won't drink red wine and every night he takes a bath that steams with the purifying fumes of an extraordinary Chinese herb that he found through the Internet.

CHAPTER FOURTEEN

Research

It is quite clear that without research new cancer treatments would not become available. There are three major forms of cancer research:

- laboratory research tries to establish the molecular basis for disease from the study and analysis of cells and tumour samples
- pharmaceutical research, carried out by the pharmaceutical industry, aims to develop new treatments for cancer
- clinical research analyses the response of patients to new treatments

These three forms of research are complementary.

Laboratory Research

Our increased understanding of the biological processes of cancer has come from work done in the laboratories of the universities and research institutes funded by charitable donation. It is thanks to this research that we are now in a position to understand the processes that control cancer and also the biological properties of tumours as compared with normal tissue.

This has been a very costly enterprise but, step by step, we are getting closer to understanding the fundamental differences between tumours and normal tissues, and how cancer grows and spreads.

In recent times we have seen the completion of the human genome project, in which every gene that makes us has been catalogued. Now science is moving away from genome-based projects which involved the identification of new genes and their relation to the causes of cancer. Instead we have turned our attention to examining the functional aspects of cells: the proteins that cells make and their interaction with each other. This has become an area of great interest because it is only through proteins that cellular processes work, and it is only by understanding these processes that we can know how cells go about their business.

Pharmaceutical Research and Drug Development

Conventional medicine requires an awesome investment from the pharmaceutical industry to reach the market. The average current cost of taking a drug from development into the market runs at about $500 million. One of the major costs in drug development is testing. The first step in this lengthy process involves testing the potentially useful drugs against panels of cells to try to understand the effects of these medicines. The next phase involves testing the drug on animals. Finally, the drug is tested on limited groups of patients.

The Natural World

It used to be that industry-based research examined natural materials, sourced from the natural world, for chemicals that might have some role in the treatment of malignancy. Field workers would trawl the rain forests and ocean depths for animals, plants and small organisms having toxic qualities that could prove useful as cancer treatments. These would be taken back to the laboratory and tested for anti-cancer effects.

Many of the drugs that we use today come from the natural world. Vincristine, which is a chemotherapy agent used to treat childhood leukaemia and many adult tumours, derives from the periwinkle plant, which is a native of Madagascar. Bleomycin, a drug used to cure testicular cancer, originates from plankton found in the seas around Japan, whilst Taxol, which is currently the biggest-selling drug in oncology and is used to treat many malignancies, originates from the pine needles of the Pacific yew tree.

The initial steps in the development of these compounds involves their purification from flora and fauna and then their testing against a panel of growing cells. Those chemicals that cause cell death or cell growth retardation in this initial testing are selected for further testing.

Animal Testing

The next stage of testing involves animals. Tumours are implanted in immuno-deficient animals – that is, animals that are unable to mount an immune response against tumours. If the tumour shrinks, then this effect will be due to the treatment itself rather than the animal's response to the tumour.

The drugs that successfully cause shrinkage of tumours in animals are then subjected to further animal testing. The dosages of the drugs are increased to far beyond that which would be given to a person and the effects on the animals recorded. Untoward side-effects can be spotted and the known toxicity of the compounds established by these processes. From this important work, drug dosages which are safe to give to humans are established. These tests are absolutely critical for the development of drugs: without them it would be impossible for new treatments to be developed. It is currently impossible to do this testing in any other way. As a result of the sacrifice of animals, drugs can be used with safety on humans.

The suffering of animals in biological testing is taken most seriously and is highly regulated by the Home Office in the UK so that the testing causes as little discomfort and pain as possible.

Clinical Research

In order to find out whether new drugs have any action in cancer treatment, patients with cancer who have gone through many other treatments are asked whether they would like to be involved in trials of new drugs on a volunteer basis. Such an investigation is called a *clinical trial*. Whilst it is unfortunately true that this initial testing may not have any benefit for the patients involved, it is terribly important for the coming generations of patients who will be affected by cancer. Without these tests new drugs cannot be developed. From the results of this first raft of tests in people, the side-effects of treatment can be established in human beings and safe dosages of the drugs can be worked out.

The next step involves further testing so that doctors can sort out which types of cancer may respond to which types of drug. On average 10,000 compounds are tested for every one compound entering clinical trial. It takes seven years of development before a new drug will become available for investigation in significant numbers of patients. It is only by this lengthy process that we can develop new drugs for cancer.

Testing continues throughout the drug's working life, and information about potential toxicities is collated by the pharmaceutical industry and put together by individual doctors, who relate their experiences to a central register.

The pharmaceutical industry, which is often criticised, has an important role to play in the development of new drugs. New drugs only occasionally come from university research programmes and almost always are the result of directed, oriented, pharmaceutical company investigations. It is with these investigations that new treatments for cancer have developed, and there have been many in recent decades.

So it can be seen that the whole process of drug develop-ment involves a massive enquiry as to safety, and this enquiry proceeds through many, many levels and continues during the drug's active life. Many drugs will have known side-effects and these are generally described to patients before they take their medicines. Occasionally drugs will be found to have surprising toxicities, such as that of Thalidomide upon the unborn child, and these side-effects are unpre-dictable. Because of the importance of drug safety, there is a very precise cataloguing of the effects of conventional medicines.

The same sort of testing is not applicable to complementary medicines, because the tests applied here are those used to investigate foodstuffs. These tests are not rigorous and require only a minimal level of safety investigation. In addition, the rigors of the processes applied to complementary medicines do not encompass any sort of scientific evaluation of efficacy. This is in direct contrast to the testing that is carried out on conventional drugs made by the pharmaceutical industry.

Quality of Life

Quality of life issues have become terribly important in modern times. Drugs which had toxicity and were used in the treatment of cancer have been refined over the years and modern equivalents have been produced that do not cause major side-effects. In the last twenty years, medicines that can control the side-effects of treatment have also been produced and these are able to minimise vomiting, reduce the problems of infection and prevent the damage to vital organs, such as the heart, that may result from chemotherapy.

Prostate Cancer Research

In prostate cancer there are a number of very important issues that require elucidation. Probably one of the most important is to try to develop new tests for prostate cancer. We know that the PSA test is a poor one in that it has a low level of accuracy in the diagnosis of malignancy because raised PSA levels also occur in benign prostatic conditions and infections of the prostate. It would be wonderful for both doctors and patients to have a new test that is much more specific to prostate cancer.

It is clear that a significant proportion of early stage prostate cancer is indolent and will not impact upon the lives of the vast majority of patients. However, there is a significant proportion of patients whose tumours, regardless of microscopic appearances, have a more aggressive character. It is not possible to distinguish between these two groups using current tests. New tests are needed to identify and segregate these aggressive tumours from indolent cancers so that necessary and better treatments can be applied.

The other big issue for patients with prostate cancer is, of course, the problem of relapse. That is, the increase in the cancer's activity after a period of response to treatment. If one could understand the biological processes that lead to this step and control them, then it might be possible for patients to live longer in some sort of peaceful equilibrium with their cancer.

Funding Research in the UK and USA

Laboratory research is funded by charitable donation and governmental agencies. Government spending in the United Kingdom on prostate cancer reached an all-time low in the financial year 1996–1997, when it is estimated that central spending through research councils was £78,000. The government has responded to recent publicity by planning an increase in spending, and it is estimated that by the year 2003–2004 central spending on prostate cancer will reach £4.3 million. This is a little below the level of spending for breast cancer, which affects a similar number of people in the United Kingdom.

In the United States, government research spending is centrally channelled through the National Cancer Institute's research programme and also through a major charity called CaPCure, the equivalent of the Prostate Cancer Charity in the UK. CaPCure was set up by the junk bond trader, Michael Milken, who, on the day of his release from imprisonment for fraud, found that he had prostate cancer. He subsequently set up a charity to sponsor prostate cancer research and in the first year had drafted all living American Presidents to support his endeavour and found $50 million to sponsor prostate cancer research.

It is through such major initiatives that science advances for people with prostate cancer and a way forward will be found to help us cure prostate cancer.

CHAPTER FIFTEEN

Screening for Prostate Cancer

It is strongly argued that a wide-ranging screening programme should be established to try to limit prostate cancer deaths. However, the issue of whether or not screening for prostate cancer will affect death rates is debated with some acrimony. Currently 1–2% of UK males and 20% of US males are screened. The impetus for this wide statistical difference is that screening is patient-driven in the UK, whereas in the United States approximately 67% of GPs accept the need for screening of their patients for possible prostate cancer.

Prostate cancer screening currently consists of the measurement of levels of the prostate specific antigen (PSA) in the bloodstream and a rectal examination. I have explained previously that PSA is a protease (an enzyme that breaks down proteins) which is made almost exclusively by the prostate and which functions in maintaining the patency of the prostatic ducts. This is a complicated way of saying that PSA is like Dyno-Rod for the prostate, cleaning out the tiny tubes that silt up with semen. PSA testing was initially approved by the American Food and Drugs Authority in 1986 for prostate cancer monitoring and in 1994 for prostate cancer screening. It is relatively non-specific as a tool for the detection of prostate cancer. It is an inaccurate and insensitive test, as PSA levels are also elevated in benign prostatic hypertrophy (BPH) and prostatitis.

There is an age-corrected normal range. In other words, PSA levels increase in normal men with age so that the normal range is different for different age groups of men. The normal PSA value for the diagnosis of prostate cancer is > 4 ng/ml. But at raised levels between 4 and 10ng/ml just 25% of patients will have prostate cancer, and at levels between 10 and 40 ng/ml only 40% will have prostatic cancer.

The lack of specificity of PSA for the early detection of prostate cancer was first described in the Physicians' Health Study published in the early 1990s, in an analysis of 22,071 male physicians who had been recruited to a prospective study. At the start of the study none of the doctors had prostate cancer. Over a ten-year period of follow-up, 520 men within this group of 22,071 men developed prostate cancer. PSA levels when measured in serum stored at the start of the study were raised in 46% of the men who developed prostate cancer. This means that in the other 54% there was no clue from PSA that a cancer was about to develop.

Refining PSA

The specificity of PSA for the detection of prostate cancer may be increased by various arcane refinements, which include *volume-corrected* PSA, PSA *velocity*, and percentage *free* PSA.

- volume corrected PSA involves a correction of the PSA value based on an estimate of the volume of the patient's prostate

- PSA velocity is a measurement of the rate of change of PSA over a period of months
- free PSA is a measure of the amount of PSA that is free in the blood and not bound to protein

It is not clear how frequently PSA should be measured, but a recent report indicates that bi-annual screening reduces mortality. Unfortunately, the bottom line in the cost-benefit analysis of such extensive testing is beyond any state funding system.

Screening in the UK

The situation with regard to screening in the UK is not clearly defined, due to the lack of specificity of PSA as a diagnostic test and the enormous expense of screening and then treating 'normal' men. Attempts have been made to screen for prostate cancer in only the relevant populations at risk and by so doing increase diagnostic specificity. However, patients at risk do not seem to be confined to specific groups. As I explained in Chapter 2, there is little evidence of a genetic basis to this disease: in a study of over 7,000 men with prostate cancer, a family history of the disease was obtained in just 159 men.

One of the reasons for the world-wide delay in the implementation of screening for prostate cancer is that it has not been proven in any randomised study that the early treatment of localised prostate cancer in patients who have no symptoms decreases death rates. So whilst the argument from the patients' hearts says 'it must be better to catch a cancer early', the rationalists reply, 'it's not been proven in prostate cancer'.

This is very similar to the situation in the 1970s when, prior to the implementation of screening for breast cancer, there were arguments about the rational basis for such a screening programme. Mammographic screening was introduced against the view of the clinicians ... and deaths from breast cancer have fallen by 30% – from 14,500 to 11,700 currently in England and Wales each year.

Despite all the clinicians' arguments against screening for prostate cancer, patients retain the connection that screening reduces death rates from this disease. The patients' view may be correct, because The European Study of Prostate Cancer Screening has recently reported a decrease in both distant and early stage disease, together with a decline in prostate cancer mortality when men are screened.

Meanwhile, in the year 2001, the UK government has announced the availability of PSA screening – on demand and with the patient's GP's agreement. We await with hope the impact of this announcement on prostate cancer mortality. We want it to fall.

CHAPTER SIXTEEN

Questions to Ask Your Doctor

Contrary to what you may read in the papers, your doctor is very likely to be trying hard to help you. You may be quite nervous in the clinic, so it's helpful to have a list of questions ready to ask. These are some suggestions.

General Questions

1. Could you explain to me the significance of my PSA levels?
2. Could you tell me about the stage and grade of the cancer?
3. Has the cancer spread?
4. What are my long-term prospects?
5. Do I need treatment at all?
6. What do you think is the best treatment for me?
7. What are my chances for a remission of my illness ... will the treatment work?
8. Are there any side-effects of treatment?
9. Are there any alternative treatments?
10. Is there any benefit from vitamins?
11. Should I change my diet?
12. Can I still drink alcohol?

Watchful Waiting

1. What are the chances that I will need treatment at some point?
2. Why don't I need treatment?
3. What are the benefits of not having active treatment?
4. When would I need treatment?
5. What symptoms should I look out for?
6. How often do you advise that I be seen for follow-up?
7. Are there any risks to this approach?
8. Does this mean that I will never be treated?
9. What are the features of my illness that indicate that no active treatment is required?

External Beam Radiotherapy

1. What are my chances of cure?
2. How long does treatment last?
3. Do you have computer planning?
4. Do you advise conformal radiotherapy?
5. What are the side-effects of treatment?
6. What proportion of patients develop impotence?
7. What percentage become incontinent?
8. Do you advise extra hormone treatment?
9. How long do you think that the additional hormone treatment should last?
10. Do you advise early treatment with Viagra for impotence?

Brachytherapy

1. (To be asked with some tact.) Is this done often in this hospital?

2. How many anaesthetics will I require?
3. Is this procedure risky?
4. Are there any immediate side-effects?
5. How long will I be in hospital?
6. Are there any long term side-effects?
7. Is there any risk of impotence, incontinence or chronic diarrhoea?
8. Will I be cured?
9. What is my chance of surviving ten years?
10. Why is this the best treatment for me?

Radical Surgery
1. (To be asked tactfully.) Do you do this operation often?
2. What are my chances of cure?
3. How long will I be in hospital?
4. How long does it take to recover from the operation?
5. How long is the catheter left in after surgery?
6. What is the likelihood of my being sexually potent after surgery?
7. What is the chance of my being continent after the operation?

Hormone Treatment
1. Do you recommend intermittent treatment?
2. Do you advise using a combination of tablets and injections?
3. How effective is treatment?
4. Is there a chance that things will get worse?
5. How long have I got?

6. Are there side-effects?
7. What are the side-effects of treatment?
8. Is there any treatment that is without side-effects?
9. What do I do about side-effects?
10. Is there any treatment for hot flushes or for impotence?
11. Are there treatments when and if the illness comes back?

Palliative Radiotherapy

1. How many treatments do you recommend?
2. Will this help my pain?
3. What are the chances that I'll get better?
4. Is there any other choice of treatment?
5. Is radioactive strontium a good idea for me?
6. Should I expect any side-effects?
7. Will I become radioactive and harm other people?

Alternative Approaches

1. Can you explain to me how this therapy/treatment works?
2. Is this therapy often used in the treatment of cancer?
3. (To the alternative practitioner or therapist.) What experience do you have of treating patients with prostate cancer?
4. In what ways do you think I will benefit from this approach?
5. Explain to the therapist/practitioner what other treatment you are receiving, and then ask, 'Is what you do compatible with the medicine/treatment I am already

receiving?' No genuine complementary therapist or practitioner will tell you to go against the advice of your doctor.

6. What sort of relief can I expect for my symptoms?

7. How many sessions do you think I need? What interval do you advise between sessions?

8. How much does a session with you cost?

9. Where can I find out more about the treatment you offer?

10. Will I feel anything during treatment? And afterwards?

11. What proof do you have that this works?

CHAPTER SEVENTEEN

Additional Information

Useful Books

Some of the books listed below are non-British and may not, therefore, accurately reflect the treatment options available in the UK. However, these books have been selected because the information contained is well written and often takes the form of a patient's account of life with prostate cancer.

Illness as a Metaphor
by Susan Sontag, published by Penguin Books

A Grief Observed
by C S Lewis, published by Faber & Faber

Dying
By John Hinton, published by Penguin Books

Prostate Problems
by Jane Smith and Dr David Gillatt, published by Hodder and Stoughton

Man to Man (American)
by Michael Korda, published by Little Brown

Living with Prostate Cancer (Canadian)
by Audrey Currie Newton, published by McClelland & Stewart Inc.

Prostate Cancer – Making Survival Decisions (American)
by Sylvian Meyer and Seymour Nash, published by The University of
Chicago Press

Understanding Cancer of the Prostate
by CancerBACUP (British Association of Cancer United Patients)
published by CancerBACUP ISBN 1-870403-71-1
Available free from BACUP (Tel: 020 7696 9003)

Understanding Prostate Disorders (Family Doctor Series)
by Professor David Kirk, published in association with the British
Medical Association (BMA)

Making the Prostate Therapy Decision (American)
by Jeff Baggish MD
published by Lowell House

Pain: the Science of Suffering
by Patrick Wall
published by Weidenfeld and Nicholson

Useful Addresses

The Prostate Cancer Charity
3 Angel Walk
Hammersmith
London W6 9HX
Tel: 020 8222 7622 (general enquiries and donations)
Fax: 020 8222 7639
Helpline: 0845 300 8383
E-mail: info@prostate-cancer.org.uk
Website: www.prostate-cancer.org.uk

The Prostate Cancer Charity was established in 1996 with the primary purpose of improving the outlook for the many thousands of

men and their families whose lives are affected by prostate cancer. The objective of the Charity is met in three ways:

1. Support and Information Service

The Support and Information Service, which benefits from the advice of medical and healthcare professionals, patients and family members, provides the following:

Helpline

The Charity funds a central telephone helpline (0845 300 8383) run by counsellors who can provide information on current thinking about prostate cancer as well as general support and clarification on any issues regarding the disease.

Networkers

The Charity has set up a nationwide network of people from all walks of life and with varying experiences of living with prostate cancer. These people – patients, partners and other family members – are happy to discuss your issues with you from their very own personal viewpoint. This service is co-ordinated from the Charity's main office.

Literature

The Charity supplies a quarterly newsletter and a booklet *Prostate Cancer – Everything You Need to Know*. The Charity also offers a smaller leaflet, *Prostate Cancer – The Facts*, which provides a quick overview of the disease, and a range of Factsheets on areas from diagnosis to treatment options.

Internet website

Many people want fast access to information. The Charity runs an award-winning website to meet this need. This is available at www.prostate-cancer.org.uk

2. Research

The Charity supports the concept that much more research is needed to improve current treatments available for prostate cancer patients. With this in mind has two approaches to its research activities.

The Prostate Cancer Group
This is a London-based team of scientists which the Charity wants to build to a group of twenty researchers. The group works closely with the Charity's Chairman and is focusing on how best to improve current therapies. Regionals are awarded to stimulate and support research around the UK.

Research Advisory Committee
Representatives from other scientific institutions from around the UK working in disciplines such as oncology, urology and radiotherapy help the Charity to decide how best to disburse grants around the UK.

3. Awareness building
The Charity has lobbied hard to draw as much attention as possible to the need to push prostate cancer higher up the political agenda and to ensure that people know of the organisation's existence and that it is here to help. Many of the Charity's supporters, men and women with personal experience of living with prostate cancer, help by talking to the media about their own experiences. The Charity's work is self-funded. No statutory assistance is received.

CancerBACUP
(British Association of Cancer United Patients)
3 Bath Place
Rivington Street
London EC2A 3JR
Tel: 020 7696 9003
Fax: 020 7613 2121 (from within London)
Freephone: 0800 18 11 99 (from outside London)
Website: www.bacup.org.uk

BACUP provides a wide range of publications on all aspects of cancers. The organisation operates a cancer information helpline where nurses can discuss treatments and what to expect from the disease. They also have a team of trained counsellors with whom an appointment can be made to discuss emotional difficulties surrounding your disease.

Cancerlink
11–21 Northdown Street
London N1 9BN
Tel: 020 7833 2818 (administration)
Fax: 020 7833 4963
Helpline: 0808 808 000
Website: cancerlink@cancerlink.org.uk

Cancerlink provides support and information on all aspects of cancer by phone, letter and publications. They also train people to set up self help groups, and produce a directory of cancer support groups across the UK.

The Impotence Association
PO Box 10296
London SW17 9WH
Helpline: 020 8767 7791
Website: www.impotence.org.uk

The Impotence Association provides information and advice about impotence through publications and a telephone helpline.

The Continence Foundation
307 Hatton Square
16 Baldwins Gardens
London EC1N 7RJ
Tel: 020 7404 6875
Fax: 020 7404 6876
Helpline: 020 7831 9831
E-mail: continence.foundation@dial.pipex.com
Website: www.continence-foundation.org.uk

The Continence Foundation provides information and advice about all aspects of incontinence through factsheets, publications and a telephone helpline.

Imperial Cancer Research Fund (ICRF)
P O Box 123
Lincoln's Inn Fields
London WC2A 3PX
Tel: 020 7242 0200
Fax: 020 7269 3101
Helpline: 0808 808 000
Website: www.icnet.uk

ICRF provide written information on cancer in the form of factsheets and brochures as well as funding research into various types of cancer.

Tenovus Cancer Information Centre
College Buildings
Courtenay Road
Splott
Cardiff CF2 2JP
Helpline: 0808 808 1010
Website: www.tenovus.org.uk

Tenovus provides support and information on any aspect of cancer. You can either telephone, write or make a personal visit to their centre.

Macmillan Cancer Relief
89 Albert Embankment
London SE1 7UQ
Tel: 020 7840 7840
Fax: 020 7840 7841
Helpline: 0845 601 6161
Website: www.macmillan.org.uk

Macmillan Cancer Relief funds specialists nurses, doctors, buildings for cancer treatment and care, grants for patients in financial difficulties and a general cancer information helpline.

Bristol Cancer Help Centre
Grove House
Cornwallis Grove
Bristol BS8 4PG
Tel: 0117 980 9500
Fax: 0117 923 9184
Helpline: 0117 980 9505
E-mail: info@bristolcancerhelp.org.uk
Website: www.bristolcancerhelp.org

The Bristol Cancer Help Centre supports patients by providing residential dietary courses.

British Society of Medical and Dental Hypnosis
17 Keppel View Road
Kimberworth
Rotherham
S Yorks S61 2AR
Tel: 01709 554 558

Access to trained therapists may be obtained through this society.

Royal London Homeopathic Hospital
60 Great Ormond Street
London WC1N 3HR
Tel: 020 7837 8833
Fax: 020 7833 7229

Consultation on homeopathic remedies may be obtained at the Royal London Homeopathic Hospital.

Glossary

Accessory sex gland a mass of glandular tissue that plays a peripheral (and not a primary) role in procreation.

Acid phosphatase an enzyme made in the prostate gland.

Acute reaching a crisis rapidly; having a short and relatively severe course; sharp; poignant.

Acute bacterial prostatitis *see* Prostatitis, bacterial, acute.

Adenoma a benign tumour in which the cells form recognisable glandular structures.

Adenomatous enlargement pertaining to the growth of adenoma.

Alkaline phosphatase an enzyme produced in the liver, the bone, and other structures.

Anaesthesia a loss of feeling or sensation. Although the term is used for loss of tactile sensibility, it is applied especially to loss of the sensation of pain, as it is induced to permit performance of surgery or other painful procedures.

General a state of unconsciousness, produced by anaesthetic agents, with absence of pain sensation over the entire body and a greater or lesser degree of muscle relaxation.

Local anaesthesia confined to one part of the body.

Spinal anaesthesia produced by injection of a local anaesthetic into the subarachnoid space around the spinal cord.

Artificial urinary sphincter a prosthesis designed to restore continence in an incontinent person by constricting the urethra.

Aspiration the removal of fluids or gases from a cavity by the application of suction.

Needle removal of cell samples with suction from a specially designed needle which is attached to a syringe.

Prostatic removal of cell and / or tissue samples from the prostate gland.

Bacteria unicellular microorganisms that may be harmful to man and may cause infection or inflammation.

Bacterial localisation tests tests devised to isolate the focus of a bacterial infection in order to appropriately treat the infection. A common test is to determine if there is bacterial infection in the prostate or the urethra.

Bacterial prostatis infection in the prostate gland caused by bacteria.

Bacteriuria the presence of bacteria in the urine.

Benign not malignant; not recurrent; favourable for recovery.

Benign prostatic hyperplasia (BPH) the non-malignant but abnormal multiplication of the number of normal cells in prostatic tissue.

Benign prostatic hypertrophy (BPH) overgrowth of the prostate due to an increase in size of its constituent cells, as opposed to hyperplasia which is the multiplication of those cells. *See also* Benign prostatic hyperplasia.

Biopsy the removal and examination, usually microscopic, of tissue from the living body which is performed to establish a precise diagnosis.

Bladder The term is often used alone to designate the urinary bladder.

Bladder catheterisation passage of a catheter into the urinary bladder.

Bladder neck contracture an abnormal narrowing of the bladder neck such that urine passage is hindered. Can be a complication of prostate surgery.

Bladder outlet the first portion of the natural channel through which urine flows when it leaves the bladder.

Bladder outlet obstruction obstruction of the bladder outlet causing problems with urination and / or the retention of urine in the bladder, *See also* Bladder outlet.

Bladder spasm a sudden and involuntary contraction of the bladder muscle(s), often attended by pain and interference with bladder function.

Bladder trigone the most dependent and most sensitive part of the bladder. Located at the base of the bladder near the bladder neck.

Blastic lesion *see* Lesions, blastic.

Bone scans (shortened form of 'scintiscan') a two-dimensional picture representing the gamma rays emitted by a radiosotope concentrated in a specific tissue of the body, in this case the bones.

Bone x-rays x-rays of the bones.

Bulbous urethra the portion of the urethra just after the membranous urethra and just before the penile urethra.

Cancer a cellular tumour, the natural course of which is fatal. Cancer cells, unlike benign tumour cells, exhibit the properties of invasion and metastases.

Carcinoma a malignant new growth made up of epithelial cells tending to infiltrate the surrounding tissues and giving rise to metastases.

Capsule the structure in which something is enclosed.

Carcinoma *see* Cancer, carcinoma.

Catheter a tubular, flexible, surgical instrument for withdrawing fluids from (or introducing fluids into) a cavity of the body, especially one for introduction into the bladder through the urethra for the withdrawal of urine.

Chlamydia a family of small spherical-shaped bacterial organisms that commonly cause infection of the urethra.

Chronic bacterial prostatitis the persistence over a long period of time of bacterial prostatitis (infection).

Computed tomography (CT) scanning the imaging technique combining x-rays with computer technology to provide a cross-section image.

Continuous or indwelling catheterisation meaning that the patient has a catheter in place in the bladder for a protracted length of time.

Contracture (bladder neck) *see* Bladder neck contracture.

Creatinine a normal metabolic waste product the measurement of which in the blood is used as an excellent parameter of kidney function.

Cystoscope an instrument used for the examination of the interior of the urinary bladder and urethra.

Cystoscopy direct visual examination of the urinary tract with a cystoscope.

Cytology the study of cells: their origin, structure, function, and pathology.

Decompensated bladder a bladder that does empty after voiding and in which residual urine remains after voiding.

Detrusor term for the smooth muscle forming the muscular wall of the urinary bladder. On contraction it serves to expel the urine.

Digital rectal examination (prostate) examination of the prostate by insertion of the finger into the rectum.

Diverticulum a pouch . . . branching out from a hollow organ structure such as the bladder.

Dribbling, terminal an involuntary loss of urine at the conclusion of voiding which occurs in drops or in an unsteady stream.

Ejaculate the semen expelled in a single ejaculation.

Ejaculatory duct the tubular passage through which the semen reaches the prostatic urethra during orgasm.

Enucleation the removal of an organ, a tumour, or another body in such a way that it comes out clean and whole, like a nut from its shell.

Enzyme-linked immuno assay a type of laboratory test in which an enzyme level is determined using an immunological assay.

Epididymis an elongated, cordlike structure along the posterior border of the testis which provides storage, transit, and maturation of sperm.

Epididymitis inflammation of the epididymis.

Epithelium the covering of internal and external surfaces of the body, including the lining of the blood vessels and other small cavities.

Erectile dysfunction impaired or disordered function of the penis regarding its role in vaginal penetration. Also called impotence.

Excretory urogram (IVP) *see* X-rays.

External urethral sphincter the ringlike band of muscle fibres that voluntarily constricts the passage of urine from the bladder to the outside.

False negative the erroneous result of a test when it is reported as negative, but it is truly positive.

False positive an erroneous report of a test as positive when it is truly negative.

Flow rate (urine) the measurement of urine as it is expelled from the bladder at is peak period of movement. If this measurement is lower than normal values, it shows that obstruction might be present.

Foley catheter a catheter which is placed into the bladder for continuous drainage and which is left in place by means of a balloon which is inflated – within the bladder – with liquid.

Frequency the desire to urinate at close intervals.

General anaesthesia *see* Anaesthesia, general.

General practitioner a family physician who treats a wide variety of medical problems, usually referring patients to appropriate specialists where indicated.

Gland an aggregation of cells, specialised to secrete or excrete materials not related to their ordinary metabolic needs.

Grading (prostatic carcinoma) the degree of malignancy, based on its microscopic appearance.

Haematuria blood in the urine.

    Gross haematuria urine in which blood is visible.

    Microhematuria urine in which blood is present, but can only be seen through microscopic examination.

Hesitancy delayed initiation of the urinary stream.

Hormonal therapy treatment through the use of hormones.

Hormones Chemicals released by glands into the blood.

Hyperplastic (prostate) tissue *see* Benign prostatic hyperplasia.

Hypertrophy *see* Benign prostatic hypertrophy.

Hytrin (terazosin) a drug used in the treatment of hypertension which is helpful in relieving the symptoms of an enlarged prostate (BPH).

Immuno-assay *see* Radioimmuno-assay.

Impotence the lack of ability of a male to initiate or maintain an erection of his penis that is sufficient for vaginal penetration.

Incontinence the inability to control the voiding of urine.

    Overflow the condition wherein the bladder retains urine after each voiding and therefore remains virtually full all or most of the time. The urine then involuntarily escapes from the full bladder by "spilling over".

    Stress involuntary discharge of urine when there is an increase in the pressure within the bladder, as in coughing or straining.

    Total failure of voluntary control of the sphincters (bladder neck and urethral) with constant or frequent involuntary passage of urine.

Indium scans *see* X-rays.

Indwelling catheterisation *see* continuous or indwelling catheterisation.

Infection invasion by pathogenic microorganisms of a bodily part in which conditions are favourable for growth, production of toxins, and resulting injury to tissue.

Inflammation redness, and / or heat, and / or swelling, and / or pain caused by irritation, injury, or infection.

Intermittent catheterisation catheterisation, usually by one's self, on a systematic interval schedule in order to be certain that the bladder is emptied of *all* urine.

Isoenzymes one of two or more chemically distinct but functionally identical forms of an enzyme.

Lateral lobes (prostate) the two paired lobes which often grow into the prostatic urethra and cause the symptoms of BPH.

Lecithin granules the granules found in prostatic secretions. They are decreased in bacterial infection in the prostate.

Lesion a wound or injury.

    Blastic refers to the increased density of bone seen on x-rays when there is extensive new bone formation due to cancerous destruction of bone.

    Lytic refers to the decreased density of bone seen on x-rays when there has been destruction of bone by cancer.

Leydig cells the cells within the testis that produce testosterone.

Lobes, prostate there are five distinct lobes of the prostate: two lateral, a middle, an anterior, and a posterior. Only the two lateral lobes and the middle lobe play a role in BPH.

    Lateral the paired lobes of the prostate which often contribute to BPH.

    Middle the commonest cause of the symptoms of BPH, the middle lobe cannot ever be felt on digital rectal examination.

Local anaesthesia *see* Anaesthesia, local.

Luteinising hormone-releasing hormone (LH-RH) a hormone which acts on the testis to stimulate testosterone production.

Lymph node Lymph nodes serve as a defense mechanism for the body by removing bacteria and other toxins. They are also a common site for cancer spread.

Lytic lesions as seen on x-rays, rarefied areas of bone that have been the site of destruction by cancer cells.

Magnetic resonance imaging (MRI) similar to CT scanning in that cross-sectional images are obtained, an entirely new methodology for imaging. There is no ionising radiation to which the patient is exposed and no known hazard to this study. It may eventually replace CT scanning as the most advanced and helpful means of imaging available.

Male hormones the hormones which are masculinising consisting of androsterone and testosterone.

Male reproductive system that part of the male concerned with the production, maturation, and transport of sperm to the outside.

Malignant tending to become progressively worse and to result in death; having the properties of invasion and metastases as applied to tumours.

Membrane a thin layer of tissue which covers a surface, lines a cavity, or divides a space.

Membranous urethra that portion of the male urethra that is within the external urethral sphincter muscle. The membranous urethra is in contact with the prostatic urethra on the bladder side with the bulbous urethra on the penile side.

Mesodermal one of the three primary layers of the embryo. The trigone of the bladder is derived from mesoderm.

Metastatic cancer cancer that has spread outside of the confines of the organ or structure in which it arose.

Metastasis the spread of disease (cancer) from one organ or structure to another or to an area removed from the original site of cancer.

Middle lobes (prostate) one of the lobes of the prostate gland, not palpable on digital rectal examination, and the lobe that is most commonly the cause of the symptoms of BPH.

Midstream (second-glass) urine the urine from the middle of the voided stream where the initial and terminal parts of the stream voided elsewhere. The middle portion of the stream is presumed to contain urine from the bladder, the ureter, or the kidney but not from any portion of the urethra or the bladder neck.

Needle aspiration of the prostate *see* Aspiration, needle.

Nocturia being awakened during the night by a desire to void.

Nonbacterial prostatis inflammation in the prostate gland in the absence of any demonstrable bacterial organisms.

Non-specific urethritis infection in the posterior urethra caused by any non-bacterial organism deleted.

Occult prostatic carcinoma a carcinoma of the prostate that is neither suspected nor diagnosed but is discovered serendipitously after prostate surgery for BPH. Also called stage A prostate cancer.

Oestrogen therapy the use of oestrogen in the palliative treatment of prostate cancer.

Oncologist a doctor who specialises in the treatment of cancer

Orchiectomy/Orchidectomy the surgical removal of both testes.

Overflow incontinence *see* Incontinence.

Peak urine flow rate the maximum rate of flow, in millilitres per second, that a patient is able to generate.

Penile prosthesis an dilatable mechanism that is inserted into the corpora cavernosa (spongy bodies) of the penis so as to make the penis rigid enough for vaginal penetration.

Penile deleted urethra urethra that is in contact with the bulbous urethra and continues all the way to the urethral meatus.

Perineal pertaining to the perineum, the area of the body between the scrotum and the anus.

Posterior urethra that portion of the urethra enclosed within the prostate gland and within the exterior urethral sphincter. These areas are known as prostatic urethra and the membranous urethra.

Primary sex gland a gland necessary for reproduction. In the male, the testis is a primary sex gland.

Proscar (Finasteride) a recently approved drug for the treatment of benign enlarged prostate (BPH).

Prostate or prostate gland a gland in the male which surrounds the neck of the bladder and the first portion of the urethra as it leaves the bladder. Its principal function is to produce the majority of the fluid in which spermatozoa travel to the outside. It also provides some of the nutrient material for the spermatozoa during their journey. The prostate is made up of connective tissue, muscle, and glandular tissue; it is the glands that manufacture the prostatic fluid.

Prostatic cancer cancer arising in the prostate.

Prostate specific antigen (PSA deleted) a protein that is manufactured in the prostate gland deleted by both benign and malignant prostate cells.

Prostate surgery

Perineal an approach to the prostate through the perineum. This approach can be used for the treatment of BPH.

Radical perineal an approach to the prostate through the perineum; this approach is used to treat prostate cancer. In this operation, the entire prostate gland is removed.

Radical retropubic an approach through the lower abdomen and behind the pubic bone that is used to treat prostate cancer. In this operation, the entire prostate gland is removed.

Retropubic an approach through the lower abdomen and behind the pubic bone that is used for the treatment of BPH. It is sometimes referred to as conservative retopubic prostatectomy.

Suprapubic an approach through the lower abdomen and through the bladder that is used to surgically treat BPH.

Transurethral a surgical approach done through the urethra to relieve the symptoms of BPH.

Prostatic adenoma *see* Adenoma.

Prostatic aspiration *see* Aspiration.

Prostatic biopsy *see* Biopsy.

Prostatic fossa *see* Fossa.

Prostatic massage a procedure whereby the index finger massages each of the two lateral lobes of the prostate for the purpose of obtaining secretions from the prostate gland. These secretions come out through the urethra.

Prostatic secretions the fluid that is manufactured in the prostate gland and obtained by means of prostatic massage.

Prostatic urethra that portion of the urethra that is enclosed within the prostate gland. It begins at the bladder neck and ends at the external urethral sphincter.

Prostatitis, bacterial, acute an inflammation of the prostate gland due to bacterial infection in which the patient is acutely ill.

Prostatitis, bacterial, chronic an inflammation of the prostate gland due to bacterial infection.

Prostatitis, nonbacterial an inflammation of the prostate gland that is not due to bacterial infection. It is presumably caused by an engorgement or statis of prostatic secretions within the prostate gland.

Prostatodynia pain in the perineal, rectal, or suprapubic area that is attributed to the prostate gland. In this condition the prostate gland is entirely normal.

Prosthesis (penile) an inflatable apparatus that is inserted into the penis to make it rigid enough to allow for vaginal penetration. It is used for patients with erectile dysfunction (impotence).

Proteinuria the presence of protein in the urine. Small amounts of protein in the urine (up to 150-200 mg per 24 hours) are normal, beyond that is considered abnormal.

Pubic symphysis the joint, formed by a union of the bodies of the pubic bones in the midline by a thick mass of fibrous, cartilaginous material. It is the hard area felt by pressing firmly on the pubic hair line.

Pyuria the presence of white blood cells in the urine.

Radical prostatectomy the radical or total removal of the entire prostate gland deleted for the treatment of prostate cancer.

Radio-immuno assay an immunological technique for the measurement of minute quantities of antigen or antibody, hormones, certain drugs and other substances found within the body.

Radioisotope an isotope which is radioactive, thereby giving it the property of decay by one or more of several processes. Radioisotopes have important diagnostic and therapeutic uses in clinical medicine and research.

Rectal examination (prostate) the insertion of an examining finger into the rectum for the purpose of feeling the prostate gland.

Renal scans (renal scanning) the production of a two-dimensional picture (the scan) representing the gamma rays emitted by a radioactive isotope concentrated in a specific tissue of the body, in this case the kidney. Renal scans are used to determine blood flow to the kidney, kidney function, and obstruction to drainage to the kidney.

Resection (transurethral) the removal of obstructing BPH prostate tissue that is done from within the urethra.

Resectoscope the instrument that is used for transurethral resection.

Residual urine any urine that is left behind in the bladder immediately after voiding. The normal residual urine is zero cc.

Retention (urinary) the inability to void when the bladder is full. This is usually caused by obstruction to the flow of urine from benign prostatic hyperplasia.

Retrograde ejaculation semen going backwards into the bladder, instead of through the urethra to the outside, during orgasm and ejaculation. This is sometimes caused by an incomplete closure of the bladder neck during orgasm and ejaculation which frequently follows transurethral resection of the prostate gland.

Retropubic the area behind and below the pubic bone and pubic symphysis.

Scans (scanning)

  Bone the production of a two-dimensional picture (a scan) representing the gamma rays emitted by a radioactive isotope concentrated in a specific tissue of the body, in this case the bone. When new bone is being laid down in a given area (a reparative phase) there is an increased uptake of the radioisotope in that area. The laying down of new bone may be in response to bone destruction from cancer spread to the bone but it may also be in response to bone trauma or even to arthritis. An increased uptake of a radioisotope in one or more bones of a patient known to have prostatic cancer strongly suggests that the cancer has spread to those bones.

Renal   *see* Renal scans.

Scrotum   the pouch or sac which contains the testes and their accessory organs.

Secretions, prostatic   the fluid that is manufactured within the many glands of the prostate gland.

Semen   the secretion of the reproductive organ in the male; it is composed of spermatozoa in their nutrient plasm, secretions from the prostate, seminal vesicles, and various other glands.

Seminal vesicle   a pouch or sac that is a paired structure and located just behind the bladder. It provides nutrient material for the spermatozoa and may store spermatozoa as well. It empties into the prostatic urethra through the ejaculatory duct at the time of orgasm and ejaculation.

Seminferous tubules   the microscopic tubules within the testis where spermatozoa are manufactured.

Sexual dysfunction   an inability to achieve or to maintain an erection, or to ejaculate would all be examples of sexual dysfunction.

Skinny-needle prostatic aspiration   the new technique by which cells from suspicious areas of the prostate are aspirated for examination. This is a form of biopsy that is becoming increasingly popular and accepted to evaluate abnormal areas of the prostate gland.

Spasm   a sudden, violent, involuntary contraction of a muscle or a group of muscles.

Spermatozoa   the mature male germ cell which is the specific output of the testes. It is the generative element of the semen, which serves to fertilise the ovum.

Sphincter (urinary)   the muscle which relaxes or contracts to control the outflow of urine from the bladder

Spinal anaesthesia   *see* Anaesthesia, spinal.

Spongy body the term for the two corpora cavernosa which are the structures within the penis that become engorged with blood during erection. When penile prostheses are used to treat individuals who are unable to achieve an erection, these paired prostheses are placed into the two corpora cavernosa of the penis so as to simulate the actual erectile process.

Staging (prostatic cancer) the process by which various tests are done to determine whether or not a prostatic cancer is still confined within the prostate gland or has spread outside of it.

Stress incontinence the inability to control the flow of urine, with resulting involuntary loss of urine, when there is an increase in intra-abdominal pressure such as occurs with sneezing or coughing.

Stricture, urethral a scarring or narrowing within the urethra that can produce symptoms of voiding difficulty very much like the symptoms of BPH. The stricture or scar within the urethra is often caused by an injury to a specific area within the urethra.

Suprapubic This is the term used for the area of the abdomen above the pubic symphysis and the pubic bone and it also refers to one of the surgical approaches for treatment of benign prostatic hyperplasia.

Surgical capsule (prostate) not a capsule at all but simply the interface between the benign prostatic hyperplasia and the true prostate gland. During surgery for the relief of BPH all of the tissue within or inside this surgical capsule is removed, leaving behind the true prostate tissue.

Testosterone the principal circulating male hormone.

Tissue a collection of similar specialised cells united in the performance of a particular function.

Trabeculation (of the bladder) the condition of the bladder muscle when it has undergone a work buildup because of obstruction to the flow of urine from BPH. The build up of the bladder muscle is irregular and induces a swiss cheese appearance within the bladder consisting of very prominent bands of built-up muscle separated by recessed areas with no apparent buildup of the muscle. The appearance of trabeculation in the bladder is strong evidence of bladder outlet obstruction, usually due to benign prostate hyperplasia (BPH).

Transurethral the route through the urethra. The term usually applies to something being passed into or through the urethra as, for example, a catheter, a cystoscope, or a resectoscope.

Trigone (bladder) the most dependent and most sensitive portion of the bladder at the base of the bladder near the bladder neck.

True capsule (prostate) the fibrous layer of tissue that surrounds the true prostate tissue.

Tru-cut biopsy needle the traditional hollow lumen needle which is used to remove a 'plug' of tissue from a solid structure (such as the prostate). It is removed for microscopic examination to determine whether or not cancer is present.

True prostate tissue the substance of the normal prostate gland. It is made up of fibrous or connective tissue, muscle tissue, and glandular tissue.

Ultrasound (ultrasonography) a technique for the visualisation of structures deep within the body by recording the echoes of ultrasonic waves directed into the tissues. Ultrasonography is a non-invasive imaging technique for detecting masses within the body and for differentiating cystic masses from solid masses. It is also used as an aid in performing biopsies of the prostate.

Uremia the retention and failure to eliminate excessive by-products of protein metabolism in the blood and the toxic condition produced thereby. It is characterised by nausea, vomiting, headache, dizziness, coma, or convulsions and, ultimately, death. The condition is usually caused by kidney failure.

Urethra the canal or channel through which urine is conveyed from the bladder to the exterior of the body. It is divided into anatomic areas beginning at the bladder neck.

Bulbous has the largest diameter of any portion of the urethra. It begins at the end of the membranous urethra and continues to the penile or pendulous portion of the urethra.

Membranous that portion of the urethra contained within the external urethral sphincter. It begins at the end of the prostatic urethra and ends at the beginning of the bulbous urethra.

Penile that portion of the urethra contained within the penis.

Posterior the term used for the prostatic urethra and the membranous urethra taken together.

Prostatic that portion of the urethra beginning at the bladder neck and ending at the external urethral sphincter. It is contained entirely within the prostate gland.

Urethral stricture an abnormal scar or narrowing at any point within the urethra. It is usually caused by an injury to the urethra.

Urethritis, nonspecific a non-bacterial infection of the urethra.

Urinary sphincter *see* Sphincter, urinary.

Urine analysis the physical, chemical, and microscopic analysis and examination of the urine.

Urine culture the incubation of urine at a specific temperature and in a specific media so as to permit the growth and identification of microorganisms. This is the definitive means by which an infection in the urinary tract is diagnosed.

Urodynamic studies quantitative means by which the two principal functions of the bladder, consisting of urine storage and urine evacuation, can be measured.

Urologist a surgeon who specialises in the surgical treatment of diseases of the urinary tract in males and females and the reproductive tract in males.

Urothelium the lining of any portion of the urinary tract.

Vas deferens the muscular, tubular structure that propels and transports spermatozoa from the epididymis into the prostatic urethra.

Weak urinary stream a voided stream that has less than normal expulsive force to it. This can be quantitated by measuring the maximum urinary flow rate expressed in millimetres per second.

X-rays electromagnetic vibrations of short wavelengths that can penetrate most substances to some extent, which are used to picture internal structures.

Index